55

CHINESE
HERBAL
SECRETS

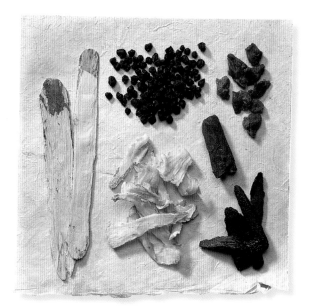

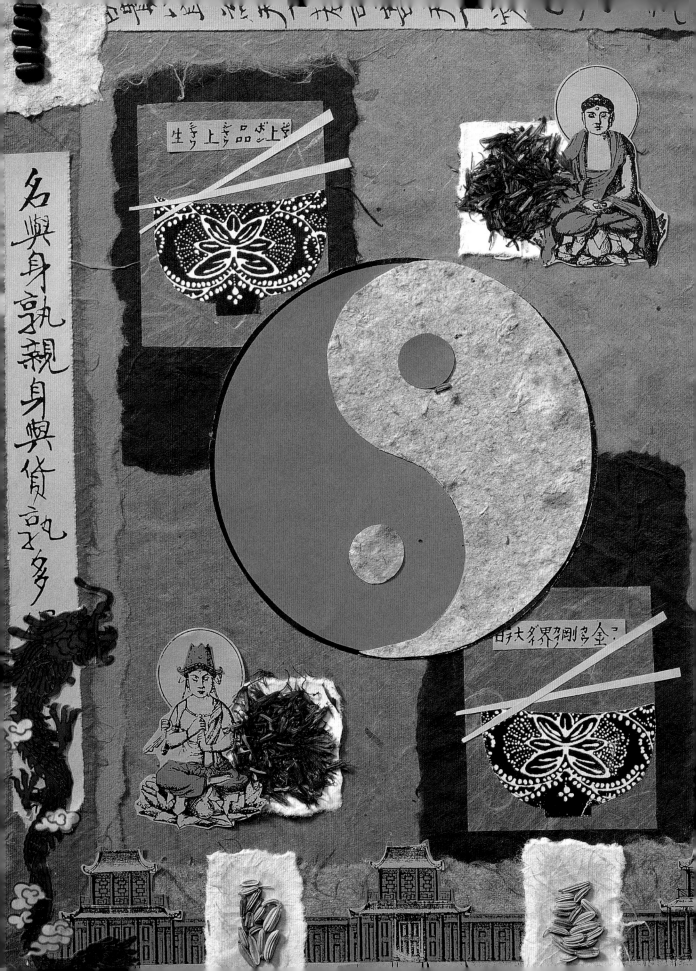

CHINESE HERBAL SECRETS

STEFAN CHMELIK

THE KEY TO TOTAL HEALTH

Newleaf

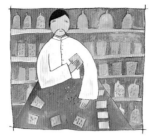

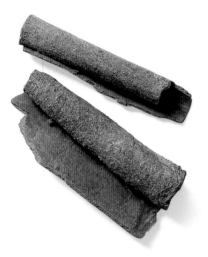

Newleaf
an imprint of
Gill & Macmillan Ltd
Hume Avenue, Park West, Dublin 12
with associated companies throughout the world
www.gillmacmillan.ie

ISBN 0 7171 3123 8

This book was conceived, designed and produced by

THE IVY PRESS LIMITED

2/3 St. Andrews Place

Lewes, East Sussex

BN7 1UP

Art director: Peter Bridgewater
Editorial director: Sophie Collins
Designer: Jane Lanaway
Senior project editor: Rowan Davies
Editor: Fiona Corbridge
Page layout: Chris Lanaway
Picture research: Vanessa Fletcher
Illustrations: Pip Adams, Pauline Allen, Michaela Blunden, Mike Courtney, Lorraine Harrison,
Andrew Kulman, Katty McMurray, Rhian Nest James
Models: Mark Jamieson
Computer graphics: Jerry Fowler
Photography: Guy Ryecart

Originated and printed by Hong Kong Graphic, Hong Kong

Cover photograph: Guy Ryecart
Frontispiece: Pip Adams

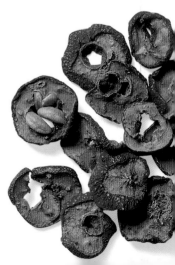

CONTENTS

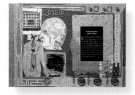

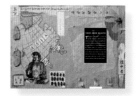

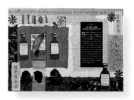

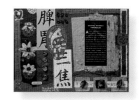

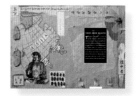

INTRODUCTION

THE QUESTION *I am most commonly asked by patients when they are interested in knowing more about me is 'how did you get involved in Chinese Medicine?'. It is a reasonable question, as for many of us Chinese Medicine is culturally specific, and people are often surprised, on meeting me for the first time, to discover that I am not actually Chinese (foreign names can be confusing, it seems).*

For me, studying this ancient system of medicine was the natural end to a process that began when I was a child. At home, the family had always been treated with non-conventional medicine, and my parents took an interest in Asian philosophies. So when I finally took the plunge and decided to study Chinese Medicine it was like coming home; I found the concepts logical, commonsensical and understandable — much more so than modern science, in fact.

I have found that this is also true with patients. Chinese Medicine provides a comprehensible framework which explains the pattern of symptoms — often seemingly random — from which people can suffer. This can be very empowering for the patient, who may be able to understand the real nature of their illness for the first time in their life.

It is my hope that this book will provide this information for you. There is a fine line between the physician's legitimate need to control access to potentially harmful procedures and substances, and the maintenance of a secrecy which is designed to shroud the profession in mystery. This is reflected by the fact that there has always been a hierarchy of treatment in China, from the 'barefoot doctor' to the court physician. Most Chinese and Asian people have a working knowledge of simple home cures, something we in the West have now largely lost. This book is designed to give some of this knowledge back to the patient while at the same time helping people to understand when to seek professional advice.

I strongly recommend that you develop a relationship with a Chinese Medicine physician even if you intend mainly to treat yourself. Regular seasonal visits to this practitioner will allow a professional to keep a general eye on what you are doing and give you the opportunity to ask questions about your self-treatment. This is also the best way to get access to the herbs you may need. A physician who is registered with the professional body for Chinese Herbal Medicine in your country will be ideally placed to know who the suppliers with the best quality control are. This is a better way of getting medicines than from unregulated small shops, where the consistency and authenticity is not controlled.

Self-treatment comes in many forms. Having to resort to medicine was traditionally regarded as something of a failure for the Chinese physician; health was maintained through the careful cultivation of good habits, and by balancing all aspects of the lifestyle. So, as well as information about herbs which treat particular conditions, this book devotes much of its content to diet, exercise and other lifestyle factors. These are areas where everybody can exert an influence on their existing and future health; the objectives are often easy to achieve, and the methods are cheap — or even free.

HOW DO I USE THIS BOOK?

Chinese philosophy and Medicine is a whole new way of looking at the world. If all of this is new to you then I recommend a traditional approach to the information in this book; start at the beginning and finish at the end. The information is presented a logical order, so that the questions raised by one section will hopefully be answered in the next. The thing I would stress most about the concepts and ideas expressed here are that they take time to understand. Simply reading all the information is unlikely to lead to a full or meaningful understanding of the concepts. It is my experience that a proper perspective and appreciation can only be reached after a certain amount of time has elapsed in study of the ideas. Take your time and enjoy yourself — read the sections as often as you like, and return to them as necessary.

SECTION ONE: DISCOVERING YOURSELF

Here you will find all the basic concepts unique to Oriental Medicine — Qi, Yin-Yang, the Five Elements, the Chinese idea of the seasons, the Eight Conditions, the Twelve Organs and the basics of self diagnosis.

SECTION TWO: HOW HERBS CAN HELP

This section introduces the problems that can be encountered in each body system and gives a number of prepared herbal remedies that can be useful in a home first aid kit.

SECTION THREE: HERBS AND THEIR PROPERTIES

The herbs are introduced and discussed in detail, broken down into categories according to their action. There are also special features on tea and ginseng.

SECTION FOUR: USEFUL HERBAL FORMULAS

This provides information about combining herbs into formulas for particular conditions. There are also food recipes for each season and sections on medicinal wines and how to make creams and ointments.

SECTION FIVE: YOUR GOOD HEALTH

The Chinese have always striven for health and longevity, and here there is information about how to apply these traditional ideas to the modern world. This section explains the environmental causes of disease and how to avoid them, and also has features on Feng Shui and healthy diet. It also includes information to expand your understanding of Chinese Medicine, such as its history and modern developments, and important guidelines on when you should consult a professional practitioner.

STEFAN CHMELIK

LONDON, NOVEMBER 1998

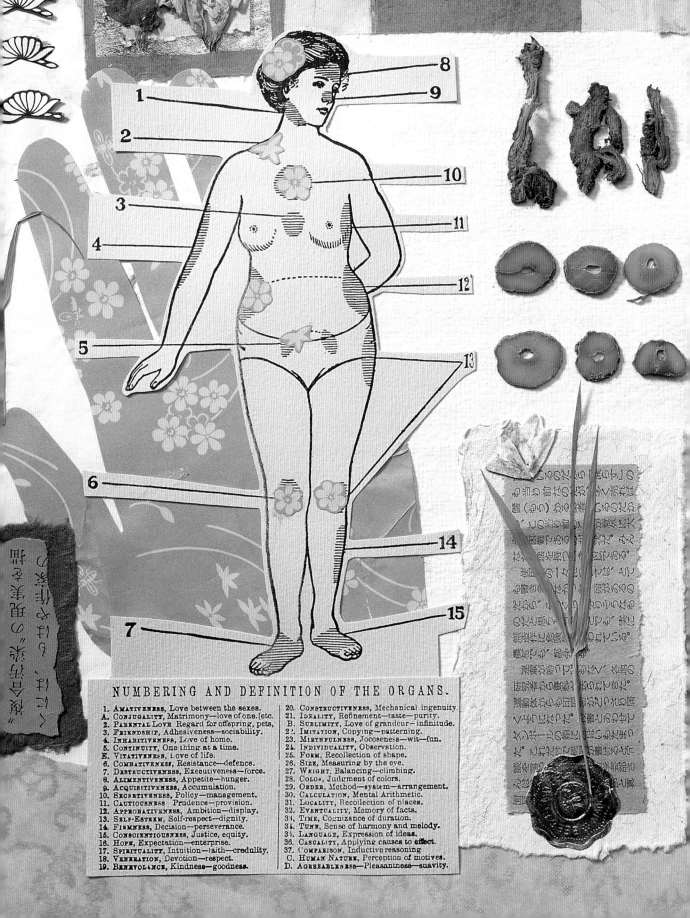

NUMBERING AND DEFINITION OF THE ORGANS.

1. AMATIVENESS, Love between the sexes.
A. CONJUGALITY, Matrimony—love of one.[etc.
2. PARENTAL LOVE Regard for offspring, pets,
3. FRIENDSHIP, Adhesiveness—sociability.
4. INHABITIVENESS, Love of home.
5. CONTINUITY, One thing at a time.
E. VITATIVENESS, Love of life.
6. COMBATIVENESS, Resistance—defence.
7. DESTRUCTIVENESS, Executiveness—force.
8. ALIMENTIVENESS, Appetite—hunger.
9. ACQUISITIVENESS, Accumulation.
10. SECRETIVENESS, Policy—management.
11. CAUTIOUSNESS Prudence—provision.
12. APPROBATIVENESS, Ambition—display.
13. SELF-ESTEEM, Self-respect—dignity.
14. FIRMNESS, Decision—perseverance.
15. CONSCIENTIOUSNESS, Justice, equity.
16. HOPE, Expectation—enterprise.
17. SPIRITUALITY, Intuition—faith—credulity.
18. VENERATION, Devotion—respect.
19. BENEVOLENCE, Kindness—goodness.

20. CONSTRUCTIVENESS, Mechanical ingenuity.
21. IDEALITY, Refinement—taste—purity.
B. SUBLIMITY, Love of grandeur—infinitude.
22. IMITATION, Copying—patterning.
23. MIRTHFULNESS, Jocoseness—wit—fun.
24. INDIVIDUALITY, Observation.
25. FORM, Recollection of shape.
26. SIZE, Measuring by the eye.
27. WEIGHT, Balancing—climbing.
28. COLOR, Judgment of colors.
29. ORDER, Method—system—arrangement.
30. CALCULATION, Mental Arithmetic.
31. LOCALITY, Recollection of places.
32. EVENTUALITY, Memory of facts.
33. TIME, Cognizance of duration.
34. TUNE, Sense of harmony and melody.
35. LANGUAGE, Expression of ideas.
36. CAUSALITY, Applying causes to effect.
37. COMPARISON, Inductive reasoning
C. HUMAN NATURE, Perception of motives.
D. AGREEABLENESS—Pleasantness—suavity.

DISCOVERING YOURSELF

Good health is so much more than merely the absence of disease. There are many people who rarely, if ever, see a doctor, but it does not automatically follow that they are healthy, in the truest sense of the word. Real health is a sense of joy and fulfilment, an appreciation of living; achieving it is entirely our own responsibility. The many different facets of our lives contribute to our overall health. Chinese Medicine looks at the big picture, showing us that health problems cannot be viewed in isolation.

This section outlines the principles behind Chinese Medicine, revealing a completely different approach to health from that of conventional Western medicine.

UNDERSTANDING CHINESE MEDICINE

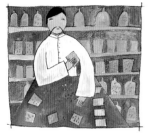

ABOVE **Thousands of herbs, in combination, are used in Traditional Chinese Medicine.**

Chinese Medicine dates back almost 5,000 years to such legendary figures as Shen Nong (the Divine Farmer) and Huang Di (the Yellow Emperor). Its basic concepts were established at a time when people lived closer to nature and the changing seasons – perhaps they were more in harmony with their surroundings than we are today. Energy flow, a close association with basic Elemental forces, and the influence of Heat and Cold, were all believed to have a great influence on well-being.

The underlying concepts

YIN AND YANG

Yin-Yang is the way in which the ancient Chinese attempted to describe the forces they could see at work in the world around them. It can be applied to all things, including the workings of the human body. The idea is that everything is based on pairs of opposing energies, with gradations between them. For example, water can be boiling hot or icy cold, with a range of temperatures between the two extremes. It is important to understand that Yin-Yang are relative concepts: a thing is only Yin or Yang in comparison to something else.

THE FIVE ELEMENTS

The Five Elements – Fire, Earth, Metal, Wood and Water – are simply another way (besides Yin-Yang) of describing natural energies. They are used to categorize the environment and to describe the body, each controlling particular organs and body functions. Each Element is associated with a flavour, colour, season, direction and many other aspects, and can be matched to body type and personality.

The Five Elements are connected in a very formal-ized way, which reflects their origination. For example, Water causes new plants to grow in spring to create Wood, which in turn is destroyed in the Fire of summer to return to ashes and Earth. Earth is the source of ores yielding Metal which, being cold, causes condensation to appear as Water.

THE TWELVE ORGANS

Each organ has a set of functions, areas of the body it controls, and a Channel or Meridian along which acupuncture points are located. These 'organs' are not to be confused with the organs of modern anatomy and Western medicine, and are generally written with a capital letter to distinguish them. The Zang or solid organs are the Liver, Heart, Spleen, Lungs and Kidneys. The Fu or hollow organs are the Gall Bladder, Small Intestine, Stomach, Large Intestine and Bladder. The other two organs are the Pericardium (the outer protective layer of the Heart), and the Triple Heater or San Jiao, which controls the distribution of Heat and Water.

QI

Qi means energy or vital force. It is the potential energy within all living things, from plants to humans. The strength of our Qi determines our vitality and is the catalyst for all the body's processes. Qi moves the Blood, and the Blood nourishes the organs in order to produce Qi. We all have different types of Qi; preserving and nurturing it is the most important step you can take to protect your health.

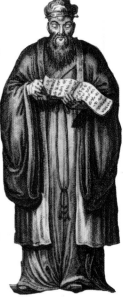

BLOOD AND
THE THREE TREASURES

The Blood represents all the moistening, nourishing, and cooling processes in the body, and works with Qi to maintain health and happiness. It nurtures the organs, especially the brain, Heart and Liver.

ABOVE **Shan Zha lowers the blood pressure and aids digestion.**

Jing or 'essence' is closely associated with inherited Qi *(see page 19),* reproductive energy and the Kidneys. As with Qi, the strength of the Jing – the energy we are born with – helps to determine our basic constitution. The Body Fluids (Jin Ye), like Blood, moisten and nourish the body, circulating from the Stomach through all the organs. Imbalance in Body Fluids is associated with Dampness and Phlegm. The Shen (Mind or Spirit) resides in the Heart, and upsets lead to insomnia, confusion and anxiety. Jing, Qi and Shen are the 'Three Treasures'.

THE EIGHT CONDITIONS

Also known as the Eight Principles, The Eight Conditions are specifically medical concepts that elaborate on the ideas behind Yin-Yang, allowing things to be defined more clearly. They are made up of four pairs of opposites: Yin-Yang, Hot-Cold, Full-Empty, Interior-Exterior. Symptoms can be defined as Full (an excess of something), Empty (a lack of something), Interior (internal causes), Exterior (external causes), Hot (diseases with symptoms of heat) or Cold (diseases with symptoms of cold). A symptom or disease can have several of these properties.

DAMPNESS AND OTHER EVILS

Illnesses result from either external causes (the Six Evils: Wind, Cold, Fire, Summer Heat, Dryness and Damp), or internal disharmony between the organs and their associated emotions, often related to imbalances in the organs' energy. The emotions are also seen as a significant cause of disease. One of the main causes of disharmony is Dampness (just like water that has leaked into the wrong place and caused damage). It happens when Fluids cease to be dealt with properly by the body, becoming thick and Stagnant. Dampness also tends to combine with any Heat that is lurking in the body, producing symptoms of inflammation. The Chinese idea of Phlegm is a further worsening of a problem caused by Damp, and this will most often be found in the Lungs.

LEFT **Confucius (551–479 BC) discussed the importance of the Five Elements in his writings.**

UNDERSTANDING THE MERIDIANS

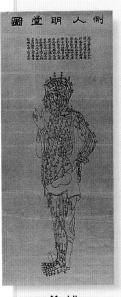

ABOVE **Meridians are associated with organs, and are used in acupuncture.**

Chinese Medicine describes a complex system of Meridians, or Channels, which are imaginary lines linking various points on the body's surface. The Meridian system distributes Qi, Blood and Fluids around the body. Each Meridian has the same therapeutic and diagnostic associations as a particular organ of the body. There are two types of Channels: the regular Channels (usually called the Jing Mai), and the small offshoots of the main Channels, called 'collaterals', or Luo Mai.

There are fourteen main Meridians: one for each of the organs, plus the governing (Du Mai) and reception (Ren Mai) vessels, which help to regulate the flow of Qi and Blood. Each of the main Meridians will have its own set of collateral Channels.

The Meridians are named after their associated organ (for example, the Lung Meridian), or after their function (as with the Conception Vessel). The Acupuncture points are sited along these Channels at varying intervals. To give an example, the Heart Meridian has only nine points, while the Urinary Bladder Meridian has 67.

Qi circulates continuously through the Channels and collaterals, and acupuncture will use the different points to stimulate or regulate this flow.

USING THIS BOOK

Chinese Herbal Secrets is divided into five parts, and is designed to make it easy for you to learn about Chinese Medicine. The book begins by introducing you to some of the important ideas and theories behind this branch of medicine, and then goes on to discuss symptoms, treatments and herbal properties in more detail.

Your five-step guide

Part One explains the basic ideas behind Chinese Medicine. Part Two discusses treatment, giving information about types of disease and their associated symptoms. Part Three gives detailed information about Chinese and Western herbs.

Part Four goes on to give combinations of herbs as formulas, enabling you to decide on a course of treatment. Finally, Part Five is devoted to more detailed information about preventative health measures, and also gives a short history of Chinese Medicine.

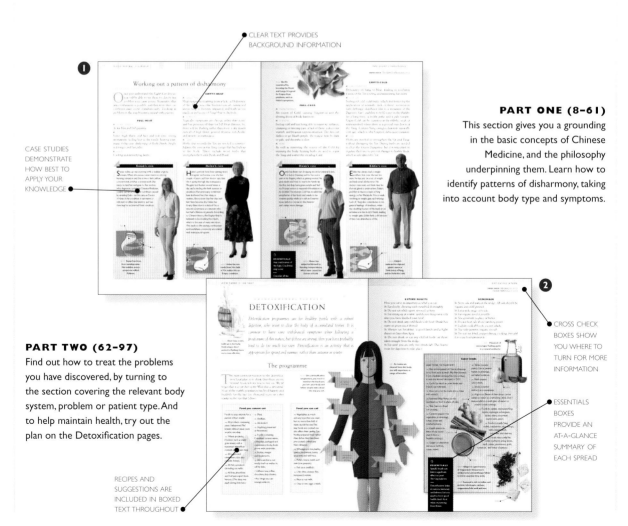

CLEAR TEXT PROVIDES
BACKGROUND INFORMATION

CASE STUDIES
DEMONSTRATE
HOW BEST TO
APPLY YOUR
KNOWLEDGE

PART ONE (8–61)
This section gives you a grounding in the basic concepts of Chinese Medicine, and the philosophy underpinning them. Learn how to identify patterns of disharmony, taking into account body type and symptoms.

CROSS CHECK
BOXES SHOW
YOU WHERE TO
TURN FOR MORE
INFORMATION

ESSENTIALS
BOXES
PROVIDE AN
AT-A-GLANCE
SUMMARY OF
EACH SPREAD

PART TWO (62–97)
Find out how to treat the problems you have discovered, by turning to the section covering the relevant body system, problem or patient type. And to help maintain health, try out the plan on the Detoxification pages.

RECIPES AND
SUGGESTIONS ARE
INCLUDED IN BOXED
TEXT THROUGHOUT

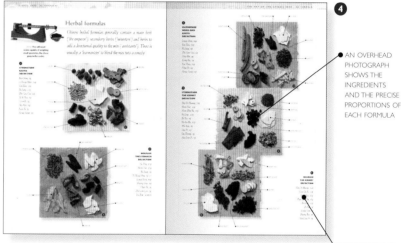

3

EACH ENTRY ALSO FEATURES A BOTANICAL ILLUSTRATION SHOWING THE HERB'S FLOWERS AND A PHOTOGRAPH OF THE PREPARED DRIED HERB

PART THREE (98–145)
This is a directory of the most useful herbs, listing their properties and the conditions treated, with recommended dosages. Herbs are grouped according to their main areas of benefit, such as those that nourish the Yin.

FOR EACH HERB, THE TEXT LISTS ROPERTIES, ACTIONS AND THE SAFE DOSAGE

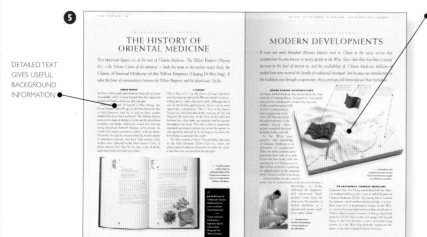

4

PART FOUR (146–165)
This section gives detailed instructions on how to make up the various herbal formulas. It also contains some delicious recipes to help rebalance the Elements, and other ways of using herbs, such as tonic wines and external preparations.

AN OVERHEAD PHOTOGRAPH SHOWS THE INGREDIENTS AND THE PRECISE PROPORTIONS OF EACH FORMULA

THE TRADITIONAL HERBAL FORMULA RECIPE IS ALSO GIVEN IN EACH CASE

5

THREE-DIMENSIONAL ILLUSTRATIONS OFFER STRONG VISUAL EXPLANATION

DETAILED TEXT GIVES USEFUL BACKGROUND INFORMATION

PART FIVE (166–175)
Here you will find a brief history of Chinese Medicine and some information about Feng Shui, plus strategies for coping better with everyday life, including a sensible exercise routine and a good diet.

THE HISTORY OF ORIENTAL MEDICINE

MODERN DEVELOPMENTS

A HOLISTIC VIEW

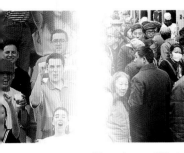

ABOVE **The cultures of West and East are very different, but we can learn much from Chinese Medicine.**

'Holistic medicine' is a term now used by millions of people all over the world. Consider for a moment what it suggests to you, bearing in mind that it is derived from the word 'wholistic'. My feeling is that to view something holistically is to look at all aspects of it at the same time. What this means for you is that each part of you – your physical, emotional and spiritual dimensions – are equally important, and imbalances in any of these areas can contribute to illness.

Holistic versus allopathic medicine

Holistic medicine considers a person's mind and body, diet and exercise, lifestyle and relationships, work and leisure, achievements and problems. You may have a pain in your leg, a headache, or be suffering from stress, but nothing can be viewed in isolation. Chinese Medicine follows this holistic principle.

However, allopathic medicine (the conventional Western method of treating illness, offered by your general practitioner) adopts a more symptomatic approach. It combats ill-health with drugs that have an oppositional effect – for example, a fever is treated with medicines to lower temperature, or painkillers are used for an aching back.

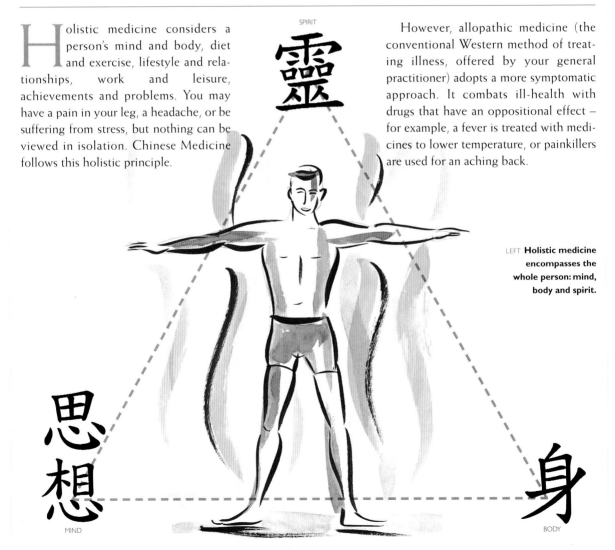

SPIRIT

靈

MIND

思
想

身

BODY

LEFT **Holistic medicine encompasses the whole person: mind, body and spirit.**

WHAT IS CHINESE MEDICINE?

Throughout this book I shall refer to Chinese Medicine as 'traditional' and conventional Western medicine as 'allopathic'. I do not consider Chinese Medicine to be either 'alternative medicine', 'non-conventional medicine', or 'complementary medicine', because it is a system of medicine that has been practised for thousands of years, like Ayurveda and Tibetan medicine, and continues to be used throughout the world. Globally speaking, these are the ancient true 'traditional' systems of medicine.

THE ALLOPATHIC APPROACH

Let's look at the case of Mr Smith, who has a stomach ulcer. An allopathic doctor would regard Mr Smith solely in terms of his disease and its symptoms, rather than as a person who happens to have a stomach ulcer. All the doctor's attention would be focused on the ulcer, rather than on poor Mr Smith.

In Chinese Medicine, however, Mr Smith's ulcer would be regarded as a reflection of a disharmony in Mr Smith as a whole. Treatment would be directed at the cause of the ulcer, such as working out why he was secreting too much stomach acid, or finding the source of the bacteria causing the ulcer.

THE CHINESE APPROACH TO ILLNESS

Chinese Medicine states that illness results when there is a disharmony in the body, or when something is out of balance. The concept of bodily organs is completely different to that of Western medicine. Organs are viewed according to their perceived functions, rather than the literal functions known to Western medicine. The twelve main organs are therefore distinguished by the use of a capital letter when referred to in Chinese terms – for example, Spleen (Chinese concept) or spleen (Western concept). This system is also used for other important organs and constituents of the body, such as the Mind and the Blood. For further information, turn to *pages 38–41.*

WHO OFFERS HOLISTIC TREATMENT?

I should stress at this point that a doctor's relative 'holisticness' is determined more by attitude than by the system of medicine practised. I have come across many allopathic doctors who truly investigate their patients' problems; likewise, there are lots of traditional (alternative) doctors who are only really performing symptom management on their patients.

LEFT **Rather like the difference between a real person and a cardboard cut-out, Chinese Medicine takes a three-dimensional approach to health, instead of viewing a problem 'flat' – in isolation.**

Two treatment systems

CHINESE	ALLOPATHIC
∽ Traditional.	∽ Conventional.
∽ Comprehensive picture of patient is painstakingly built up by the doctor.	∽ Patient is likely to be viewed solely in terms of his or her disease.
∽ Treats the whole person, not just the symptoms of the disease.	∽ Will usually consider only the disease symptoms, not the whole person.

ESSENTIALS
Ill-health is a result of imbalance or disharmony in the individual, and is not necessarily physical.

—

Chinese Medicine's holistic approach goes far beyond the physiology of Western medicine.

Chinese Medicine has been practised for several thousand years. The very nature of the Taoist principles on which it is based stresses the oneness of everything, the inseparability of solid matter and energy, and the fact that there is a common source of all phenomena and experience. The Chinese say that 'the enlightened person eats when hungry and sleeps when tired'. This means living in harmony with the energy of the seasons and with the particular requirements of your mind and body, which empowers you to influence your own health destiny.

QI ~ THE LIFE FORCE

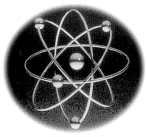

ABOVE **Like the atom in science, Qi underlies everything in life.**

Qi (pronounced 'chee') is the universal life force. It exists in the body in various forms. When our Qi is in harmony, we enhance and preserve not just our health, but also our capacity for fulfilment, happiness and well-being. Qi is responsible for all processes in the body – acting as a catalyst for metabolic change – as well as for transformations in energy states, which affect our Mind and Spirit.

Your personal needs

We all need to work at keeping our Qi in top condition for maximum health benefits. This may involve making alterations to our lifestyle, or taking herbs to cure a disharmony (ill-health). There is no such thing as a 'good' herb – a particular herb is only good for you if it is the one you need. Ginseng and Echinacea, for example, are both powerful herbs with strong medicinal actions that may be used to rectify an imbalance, but only if you have the imbalance for which they are intended.

Equally, we should remember that although we all have varying requirements, there are certain laws of nature that cannot be broken without subsequent consequences for our mental or physical health. These concern the necessity to pay attention to sleeping, eating, breathing and exercising properly.

Qi boosters

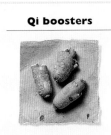

Ginseng is valued for invigorating Qi. It is one of the most expensive herbs.

Echinacea is a Western herb that stimulates the immune system and has an anti-inflammatory action.

LEFT **We all need to take as much care as we can of our internal energy – Qi.**

RIGHT **Our Qi affects health and happiness. If Qi gets out of balance, problems result.**

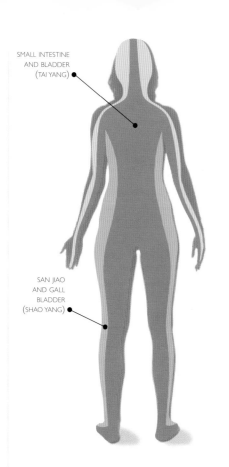

SMALL INTESTINE
AND BLADDER
(TAI YANG)

SAN JIAO
AND GALL
BLADDER
(SHAO YANG)

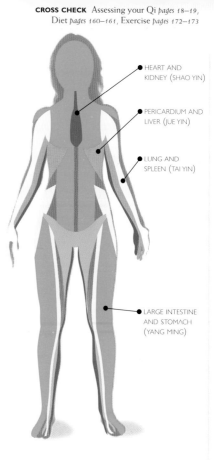

HEART AND
KIDNEY (SHAO YIN)

PERICARDIUM AND
LIVER (JUE YIN)

LUNG AND
SPLEEN (TAI YIN)

LARGE INTESTINE
AND STOMACH
(YANG MING)

ESSENTIALS
Healthy Qi results from a healthy lifestyle with the right amount of sleep, exercise, food and good breathing.

—

All these factors must be kept in balance — too much or too little of any can lead to ill-health.

LEFT AND RIGHT **The Meridian areas of the body, back and front views. Problems in an organ can be treated through its associated Meridian.**

SLEEPING

Everybody needs eight or more hours' sleep. If you consistently feel tired when you wake up, then you need more sleep than you are getting. It's just as important when those eight hours are. Essentially, human beings are designed to be asleep between the hours of midnight and 6am, with an hour or so either side for pre-sleep and post-sleep. Proper deep sleep only occurs between these hours and it is the time when the body makes vital repairs. Catnaps in the afternoon are a good way of topping up your sleep if the demands on your energy are very high, or if you are recovering from an illness.

EATING

Eating is not optional! Human metabolism is relatively constant and only altered by extremes of weather or environmental conditions. Our digestive systems work most efficiently during the early parts of the day. So the largest meals should be eaten for breakfast and lunch, and only light food eaten in the evening. This is, of course, precisely the opposite of what most of us do! Many herbal preparations are also designed to be taken first thing in the morning to utilize digestive energy. Food eaten late at night may Stagnate.

Breakfast is golden, lunch is silver and dinner is poison.

BREATHING

Sedentary jobs, lack of proper exercise, the quality of the air we breathe, and poor posture all contribute to poor breathing habits. In women, in particular, there may be a tendency to 'hold the stomach in', which prevents the diaphragm from being properly used. The diaphragm (a muscle that lies horizontally across the floor of the ribcage) controls breathing, not the ribs or the lungs. If this is not utilized, not only are the lungs never fully filled or emptied, but the organs in the abdomen are deprived of essential massage from the rhythmic action of respiration.

EXERCISE

What is the right kind of exercise? This will depend on your sex, age and constitution. Vigorous aerobic exercise is more appropriate in the first third of life, during middle age we should incorporate harmonizing and regulating pursuits, and in old age we should focus on more meditative and relaxing exercise. Your physique will also determine the amount and type of exercise that is suitable. If you have a particular weakness, you can focus gentle exercise on that area. If you are frail or recovering from illness, it is important not to deplete your resources through over-exertion.

ASSESSING YOUR QI

Knowing about your own unique resources of Qi is central to the idea of understanding your health. Chinese Medicine categorizes a person's Qi in three ways: parental Qi, acquired Qi, and inherited Qi. Some people may be blessed with strong energy resources inherited from their parents at birth. Others will need to work hard to boost their inherent energy levels by a healthy diet and lifestyle, and avoiding toxins and pollutants, which can damage Qi.

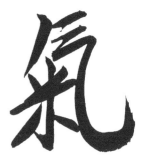

ABOVE **The Chinese brush calligraphy for Qi.**

The three types of Qi

The three basic types of Qi are parental, acquired, and inherited Qi. The original Qi received from our parents is also known as 'pre-natal' Qi; the Qi acquired during life may be described as 'post-natal' Qi.

BELOW **Although some Qi is inherited from our family, Qi can be gained or dissipated throughout life.**

PARENTAL QI

Parental Qi is the basic health you are given at birth by your parents. It is determined by your parents' state of health at around the time of (and particularly at the moment of) conception, and by the mother's health during pregnancy and labour. This correlates directly with modern research. It is known that the sperm of men who drink heavily, smoke or who are under severe stress is of a lower quality. We also know that the health of a baby can be affected by drugs taken by the mother, by her lifestyle, or by trauma during pregnancy.

ACQUIRED QI

Acquired Qi is the energy derived from the things we consume after we are born: food, fluids and air. Poor diet, excessive alcohol consumption or polluted air can contribute to bad health, even in those with strong parental Qi who are born hearty.

INHERITED QI

Inherited Qi is the essential you. It is largely determined by the general constitution of your family, and explains why certain conditions can run in a family, even if they may sometimes skip a generation.

Your Qi account

Qi can be viewed rather like money: something you spend, save or invest. To continue this metaphor, think of Qi as representing different types of bank account.

PARENTAL QI – THE DEPOSIT ACCOUNT
The deposit account can be used occasionally for special things, and to fall back on in times of emergency. It can be added to from a surplus in the current account. You get a reasonable 'interest' rate if you don't need to draw on funds very often. If this account is consistently overdrawn, you will need to fall back on your inheritance nest-egg to survive.

ACQUIRED QI – THE CURRENT ACCOUNT
The current account covers day-to-day living expenses. It will fluctuate according to your needs and the time of year. It can be depleted and renewed frequently. If you keep 'overspending' and this account is consistently in the red, you will have to keep drawing from your deposit account.

INHERITED QI – THE INHERITANCE NEST-EGG
The nest-egg is a one-off lump sum that cannot be substantially added to, and once it is used up you are broke. Sometimes people can be born with a poor inheritance, such as those who suffer from congenital illness. With time, this basic store of Qi gradually erodes. In Chinese Medicine, some natural aspects of ageing, such as the menopause, may be related to the gradual depletion of Qi.

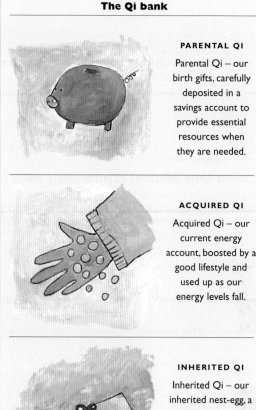

The Qi bank

PARENTAL QI
Parental Qi – our birth gifts, carefully deposited in a savings account to provide essential resources when they are needed.

ACQUIRED QI
Acquired Qi – our current energy account, boosted by a good lifestyle and used up as our energy levels fall.

INHERITED QI
Inherited Qi – our inherited nest-egg, a one-off store whose amount will vary with each individual.

Good Qi management

By eating properly, resting and exercising, you will keep your Qi current account in the black. Over a period of time this will lead to a surplus, which can be siphoned off into a Qi deposit account. If left untouched, the Qi deposit account will grow.

Work out the relative strengths and weaknesses of your Qi finances. Use this to decide which areas of your health maintenance need special attention. Nurturing Qi during the good times will increase your basic store of Qi, providing the energy resources to combat disease.

ESSENTIALS
We can do little to change our inherited Qi, but acquiring Qi will strengthen our overall energy levels.

Parental Qi largely depends on the health and well-being of our parents.

As an example, let's consider two financial situations, and draw parallels with Qi management. Adam, a trust-fund beneficiary, never needs to work at preserving Qi. Such people often do not value the Qi they have, and only realize its importance when most of it is gone. Janet, a self-made person, has not been given much to start with, but through a combination of patience, application and luck has managed to acquire a vast empire of Qi. Adam can do little to renew his energy resources, but Janet's lifetime of effort may see her outlast Adam.

YIN AND YANG

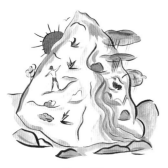

ABOVE **Yin and Yang are opposites, yet attached – like the sunny and shady sides of a mountain.**

Yin and Yang is perhaps the most well-known, but most misunderstood concept in Eastern philosophy. Some people will have an idea of what is Yin and what is Yang, although they may not be sure which way round! Well, abandon all your preconceptions now, because Yin and Yang are not about lists of 'things', nor are they separate concepts. They cannot exist in isolation, and everything contains aspects of both Yin and Yang.

The philosophy

The first recorded reference to Yin and Yang is in the *Yi Jing*, or *Book of Changes* (often written as *I Ching*), used by the Chinese for divination. Some have said that one cannot understand Chinese Medicine without studying the *Yi Jing*.

The Chinese characters for Yin-Yang describe two sides of a mountain: the sunny side, which is the Yang side, and the shady side, which is the Yin side. So this single object, the mountain, can be either Yin or Yang, dark or light, hot or cold, depending on the forces acting on it. Yin-Yang describes a relative state of transition. In other words, something is never just Yin or Yang, but is constantly in flux between the two states, and there is always a part of one in the other.

In the Yin-Yang symbol, this is represented by the dynamic curve and the contrasting dot. The line separating the Yin and Yang is not straight, but curved. This is important as it demonstrates the gradual transformation from one state to the other, and it is only at the tip of the helix that a total state of Yin or Yang exists, and then only for a moment in time.

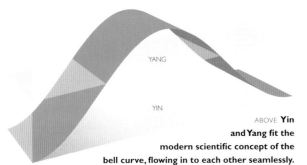

YANG

YIN

ABOVE **Yin and Yang fit the modern scientific concept of the bell curve, flowing in to each other seamlessly.**

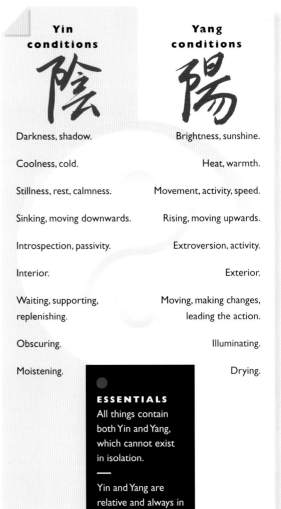

Yin conditions	Yang conditions
陰	陽
Darkness, shadow.	Brightness, sunshine.
Coolness, cold.	Heat, warmth.
Stillness, rest, calmness.	Movement, activity, speed.
Sinking, moving downwards.	Rising, moving upwards.
Introspection, passivity.	Extroversion, activity.
Interior.	Exterior.
Waiting, supporting, replenishing.	Moving, making changes, leading the action.
Obscuring.	Illuminating.
Moistening.	Drying.

ESSENTIALS
All things contain both Yin and Yang, which cannot exist in isolation.

—

Yin and Yang are relative and always in transition. Things always retain some degree of both.

The power of the moment

Although we can make certain statements about what is Yin and what is Yang, they are only snapshots in time. For example, the Chinese say that midnight is the time of absolute Yin, but midnight is not really a time – it is a transitional state between 'before-midnight' and 'after-midnight'.

Equally, when we say that hot is a Yang condition, this is only true when it is compared to something that is colder than the thing we are describing. So, a cup of hot water is Yang compared to cold tap water, but it is Yin compared to the heat emanating from a kettle that has just been boiled.

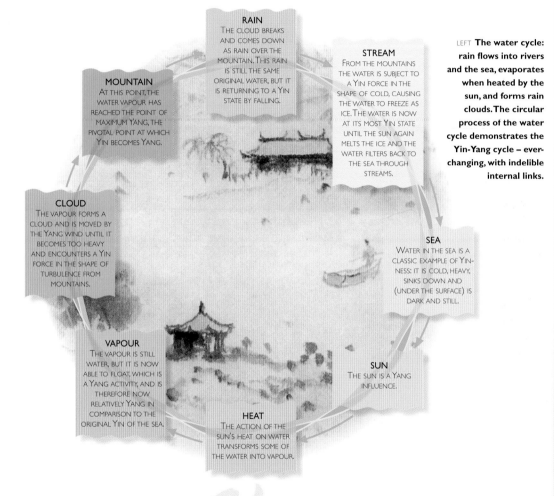

RAIN
THE CLOUD BREAKS AND COMES DOWN AS RAIN OVER THE MOUNTAIN. THIS RAIN IS STILL THE SAME ORIGINAL WATER, BUT IT IS RETURNING TO A YIN STATE BY FALLING.

STREAM
FROM THE MOUNTAINS THE WATER IS SUBJECT TO A YIN FORCE IN THE SHAPE OF COLD, CAUSING THE WATER TO FREEZE AS ICE. THE WATER IS NOW AT ITS MOST YIN STATE UNTIL THE SUN AGAIN MELTS THE ICE AND THE WATER FILTERS BACK TO THE SEA THROUGH STREAMS.

MOUNTAIN
AT THIS POINT, THE WATER VAPOUR HAS REACHED THE POINT OF MAXIMUM YANG, THE PIVOTAL POINT AT WHICH YIN BECOMES YANG.

LEFT **The water cycle: rain flows into rivers and the sea, evaporates when heated by the sun, and forms rain clouds. The circular process of the water cycle demonstrates the Yin-Yang cycle – ever-changing, with indelible internal links.**

CLOUD
THE VAPOUR FORMS A CLOUD AND IS MOVED BY THE YANG WIND UNTIL IT BECOMES TOO HEAVY AND ENCOUNTERS A YIN FORCE IN THE SHAPE OF TURBULENCE FROM MOUNTAINS.

SEA
WATER IN THE SEA IS A CLASSIC EXAMPLE OF YIN-NESS: IT IS COLD, HEAVY, SINKS DOWN AND (UNDER THE SURFACE) IS DARK AND STILL.

VAPOUR
THE VAPOUR IS STILL WATER, BUT IT IS NOW ABLE TO FLOAT, WHICH IS A YANG ACTIVITY, AND IS THEREFORE NOW RELATIVELY YANG IN COMPARISON TO THE ORIGINAL YIN OF THE SEA.

SUN
THE SUN IS A YANG INFLUENCE.

HEAT
THE ACTION OF THE SUN'S HEAT ON WATER TRANSFORMS SOME OF THE WATER INTO VAPOUR.

Balancing Yin and Yang

People are classified as Yin or Yang, depending on their personal characteristics. Yin and Yang are both essential for balance: neither is superior to the other. It is not better to be either a Yin or a Yang person, but we should strive for balance within our innate character by emulating the qualities of our opposite type. As we age, any imbalance becomes more pronounced, so that a Yang person will tend to lack Yin and will need to actively encourage Yin qualities to maintain balance – and vice versa.

Let's translate this into terms that relate to our bodies. During the day we are awake (Yang) and at night we are asleep (Yin). But there is a period when we are going to sleep and when we are waking from sleep. These are transitional states.

Somebody who feels the cold could be described as Yin, while a person who gets hot easily may be predominantly Yang. If you are tired all the time, this could be because of insufficient Yang (activity); hyperactive people may have too little Yin (stillness).

THE FIVE ELEMENTS AND THEIR ASSOCIATIONS

The Five Elements (Wu Xing) are, together with Yin-Yang, the basic 'building blocks' of the Chinese universe. They are: Earth, Metal, Water, Wood and Fire. The principles of the Five Elements can be applied to everything. Each Element is related to the world around it, with an affiliated season, colour, taste, body organ and sensory organ.

Relationships between the Elements

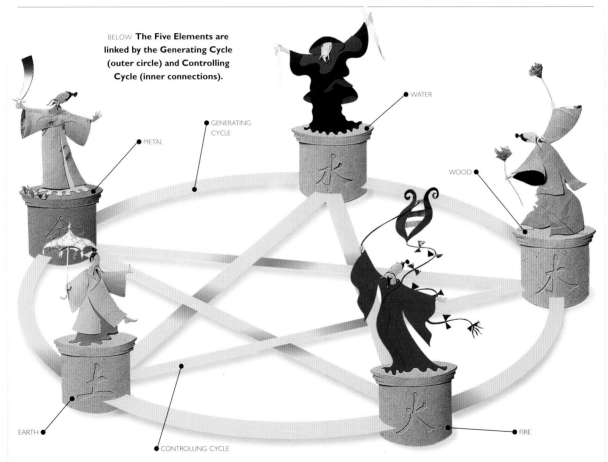

BELOW **The Five Elements are linked by the Generating Cycle (outer circle) and Controlling Cycle (inner connections).**

METAL · GENERATING CYCLE · WATER · WOOD · EARTH · CONTROLLING CYCLE · FIRE

THE GENERATING CYCLE

The Elements are about cycles and patterns of change, and are related to each other. The outer circle joining them together is called the Generating Cycle, likened to the relationship between a mother and child. That is to say, each Element generates the next Element that follows, working in a clockwise direction. For example, Water generates Wood, for without moisture there cannot be growth. Wood is the fuel to create Fire, and it is the action of heat on organic matter that produces Earth (think of a compost heap). Metal and minerals are generated from the Earth, and these filter and purify the Water that returns to feed the trees. So the cycle continues.

THE CONTROLLING CYCLE AND THE PROPERTIES OF THE ELEMENTS

The internal links between the Elements are referred to as the Controlling Cycle. This balances the Generating Cycle and explains the connections between the Elements. For example, Water will keep Fire in check and Fire can make Metal usable. The hardness of Metal is required to tame Wood. Without the controlling structure of roots, the Earth would collapse and be in disarray. Water is without shape and will always sink to the lowest level: it is Earth that defines its outline. In terms of bodily functions, this is expressed through the organ relationships between each of the Five Elements. Each Element has an associated Yin and Yang organ.

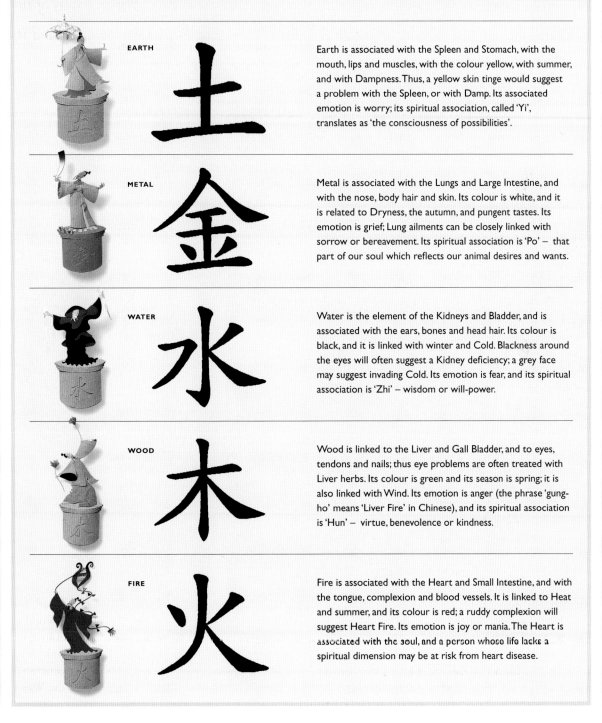

EARTH

Earth is associated with the Spleen and Stomach, with the mouth, lips and muscles, with the colour yellow, with summer, and with Dampness. Thus, a yellow skin tinge would suggest a problem with the Spleen, or with Damp. Its associated emotion is worry; its spiritual association, called 'Yi', translates as 'the consciousness of possibilities'.

METAL

Metal is associated with the Lungs and Large Intestine, and with the nose, body hair and skin. Its colour is white, and it is related to Dryness, the autumn, and pungent tastes. Its emotion is grief; Lung ailments can be closely linked with sorrow or bereavement. Its spiritual association is 'Po' – that part of our soul which reflects our animal desires and wants.

WATER

Water is the element of the Kidneys and Bladder, and is associated with the ears, bones and head hair. Its colour is black, and it is linked with winter and Cold. Blackness around the eyes will often suggest a Kidney deficiency; a grey face may suggest invading Cold. Its emotion is fear, and its spiritual association is 'Zhi' – wisdom or will-power.

WOOD

Wood is linked to the Liver and Gall Bladder, and to eyes, tendons and nails; thus eye problems are often treated with Liver herbs. Its colour is green and its season is spring; it is also linked with Wind. Its emotion is anger (the phrase 'gung-ho' means 'Liver Fire' in Chinese), and its spiritual association is 'Hun' – virtue, benevolence or kindness.

FIRE

Fire is associated with the Heart and Small Intestine, and with the tongue, complexion and blood vessels. It is linked to Heat and summer, and its colour is red; a ruddy complexion will suggest Heart Fire. Its emotion is joy or mania. The Heart is associated with the soul, and a person whose life lacks a spiritual dimension may be at risk from heart disease.

FINDING YOUR ELEMENT

We use the phrase 'in your element' to describe ourselves in peak form. In Chinese Medicine, too, we belong to a particular Element, and being in harmony with it keeps body and mind in optimum health. Refer to the likely health problems listed for each Element, and see how to counter them by herbs, diet, exercise and other methods.

THE BODY PICTURE

Historically, Chinese Medicine was based on observations of the complex processes of the human body. Over the centuries, Chinese doctors put together a system to describe human physiology, based on the principles of Yin-Yang and the Five Elements. The system made use of metaphor, allegory and even poetry to explain the functions that were observed. Much of the workings of the body were described in relation to the preoccupations of the day, so there was a lot of agricultural imagery. The flow of energy was likened to the flow of water through the land, with streams, rivers and seas being located around the body. The organs were variously described as being similar to the Emperor and his court officials, or like the workings of a kitchen. The body in general was seen as a landscape, from the Lungs as clouds above, down to the Intestines as irrigation and drainage ditches. The Five Elements all have associated organs. Their characteristics also enable us to categorize ourselves as Elemental types.

THE FIVE ELEMENTAL BODY TYPES

We all have an Element that describes the dominant aspect of our personality. We also have facets of all the Elements in our make-up, to varying degrees. It may be immediately obvious to you which Element you are, or you may not feel an affinity with any of them. This is precisely why the Chinese have developed a number of ways of defining people and diseases, and different people will be comfortable with the different systems available in this book.

Use the information on *page 25* and on the following pages to work out your Element. Introductory text describes the general flavour of the Element and its particularities. This is followed by affinities, key words, likely health problems, key herbs, foods to include and avoid, and strategies to follow.

AFFINITIES
Strong or weak points for the Elemental type. The colour that may be observed in the face or the tone heard in the voice; environmental conditions that the person will be sensitive to.

KEY WORDS
Associations that are traditionally linked to the Element in Chinese Medicine.

PRONE TO
Health problems that the Elemental type is more likely to suffer from.

KEY HERBS
Main herbs that are of benefit.

RECOMMENDED FOODS
The best foods for preserving the health of this particular Elemental type.

FOODS TO AVOID
Foods that deplete the energy of the Elemental type, and tend to cause health problems.

CULTIVATE
Ideas to consider adopting as a means of counteracting any negative qualities of the dominant Element.

Earth

土 Earth is the centre around which the other Elements revolve, much as the Earth organs of the Stomach and Spleen are the centre of the body. All nourishment comes from Earth: trees are rooted in it, and Water is filtered through its soil. Earth is a force that allows growth and development. The food and fluids we consume are processed by the Stomach to produce our Qi and Blood. The nature of an Earth person is abundance and generosity, and this bountiful attitude will often extend to taking on the cares and worries of others – sometimes excessively so.

For Earth to be productive and fertile it must be neither parched nor muddy. It is said that the Spleen likes to be warm and dry and the Stomach cool and wet. If these conditions are changed, disharmonies will result in the organs, so balance is important.

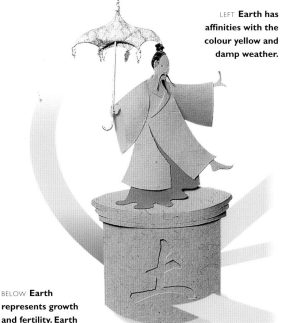

LEFT **Earth has affinities with the colour yellow and damp weather.**

BELOW **Earth represents growth and fertility. Earth people are warm and generous.**

Which Element are you? Earth

AFFINITIES
Spleen and Stomach, change of seasons, sweet tastes, the muscles and the lips/mouth, the colour yellow, a childlike voice, damp weather and damp conditions.

KEY WORDS
Nurture, nourish, transform, sympathy, worry, mothering, obsessive, oppressive.

PRONE TO
Tiredness, poor muscle tone and flabbiness, easy bruising, varicose veins, pale sallow complexion, digestive and bowel problems, eating disorders, yeast infections and food intolerance, poor memory and concentration, worry.

KEY HERBS
Ren Shen, Fu Ling, Bai Zhu, Yi Yi Ren, Shan Yao, Dang Shen, Chen Pi, Hou Xiang, Sha Ren.

RECOMMENDED FOODS
Grains such as rice and barley; naturally sweet vegetables such as carrots, parsnips, swede and squash; orchard fruits such as red apples and pears; warm spices such as ginger, garlic and cardamom.

FOODS TO AVOID
Sweet foods that include processed sugars and (especially) artificial sweeteners; an excess of tropical fruit such as bananas and mangoes; large quantities of fruit juice; too much cold fluid, especially with food; dairy products originating from cows; wheat, especially white bread.

CULTIVATE
• A liking for breakfast: it is the most important meal of the day.

• An early dinner. Do not eat late and then go to bed. Eat until only two-thirds full.

• Aerobic muscle-toning exercise.

25

Metal

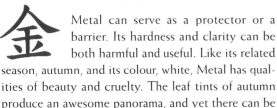

Metal can serve as a protector or a barrier. Its hardness and clarity can be both harmful and useful. Like its related season, autumn, and its colour, white, Metal has qualities of beauty and cruelty. The leaf tints of autumn produce an awesome panorama, and yet there can be a bleakness that is cold and isolating.

The Lungs and Large Intestine are associated with Metal. These organs of elimination remove waste from the body through the bowels and the skin. The skin is our external barrier, defining where we end and the outside world begins. One of Metal's functions is to protect against invasion by harmful influences, but, if it is working too efficiently, it can translate into an isolation from human contact.

Autumn is the time of death, when things return to the Earth. Grief is said to damage the Lungs, wasting them like a withering leaf. Metal is concerned with correct behaviour, protocol and virtue, and the Metal type is quick to respond to perceived injustices and injuries. Metal is cold and brittle and can lead to insensitivity. Metal people need to work at developing the spiritual side of their lives as, in a holistic approach, neglecting it can lead to physical illness. Their tendency to put up boundaries can also negatively affect their health.

LEFT **Metal is a barrier to help protect the body from harmful influences.**

BELOW **The hard-edged beauty of stalactites, and their isolation underground, echo the qualities of Metal.**

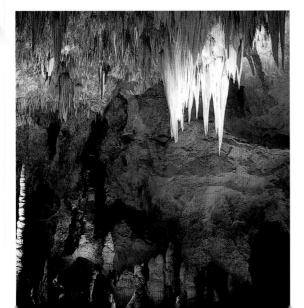

Which Element are you? Metal

AFFINITIES
Lungs and Large Intestine, autumn, pungent or aromatic tastes, the skin, body hair, the nose and smell, the colour white, a crying voice, dry weather and dry conditions.

KEY WORDS
Protection, boundaries, elimination, death, precision, isolation, sadness.

PRONE TO
Colds, airborne allergens, selfishness, coughs, asthma, dry skin, constipation.

KEY HERBS
Huang Qi, Dang Shen, Mai Men Dong, Bai He, Chen Pi, Bei Mu, Huang Qin, Sheng Jiang.

RECOMMENDED FOODS
Grains, root vegetables, pears, nuts and seeds, and some pungent spices such as ginger and black pepper.

FOODS TO AVOID
Too much baked or barbecued food, smoked food, too much dairy produce.

CULTIVATE
• A regular aerobic exercise routine.

• Your spiritual side.

• Tolerance of the weaknesses of others.

Water

水 Water is unique amongst the Elements in its ability to be everywhere yet nowhere. Water is formless, yet it takes on the form of the vessel that contains it. Water is the deep, hidden aspect within all living things.

The Water organs of the Kidneys and Bladder have an obvious role to play in the process of Water metabolism. Water also refers to the deepest aspects of growth that take place in the recesses of the Earth. Water is responsible for the bodily functions of fertility and development, and so it is Water that determines the characteristics and qualities that will be handed down to you from your parents. The strength and development of the deepest parts of the body, such as the bones, is determined by Water energy; the teeth, too, rely on it.

Water types can be isolated by their inner nature, and this can cause fearfulness about what the future will bring. The Kidneys are said to be the root of all Yin and Yang in the body, and prolonged extremes of Heat or Cold will affect Water in adverse ways, leading to a Deficiency of either Yin or Yang.

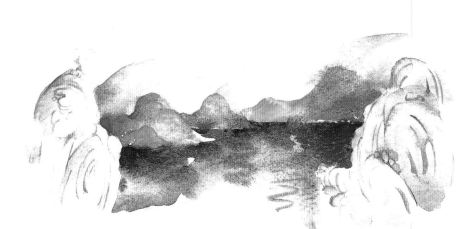

ABOVE **Water mirrors the deeper, hidden aspects of self.**

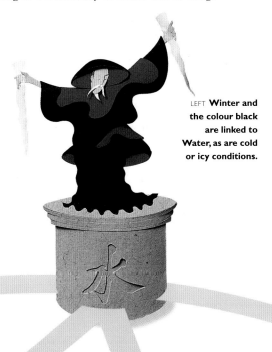

LEFT **Winter and the colour black are linked to Water, as are cold or icy conditions.**

Which Element are you? Water

AFFINITIES
Kidneys and Bladder, winter, storage, a salty taste, the bones, teeth and ears, hearing, the colour black, a groaning voice, cold weather and cold conditions.

KEY WORDS
Wisdom, destiny, will-power, constitution, development, motivation, fear, shock.

PRONE TO
Back problems, bladder problems, weak bones or teeth, hormonal changes, poor development.

KEY HERBS
Shu Di, Gou Qi Zi, He Shou Wu, Gui Pi, Du Zhong, Huang Bai.

RECOMMENDED FOODS
Seaweed, naturally salty food such as fennel and celery, warm fluids.

FOODS TO AVOID
Cold foods and fluids, excessive salt.

CULTIVATE
• An exercise routine that will keep the knees and back strong.

• A moderate love life.

• The correct fluid intake: neither too much nor too little.

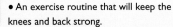

Wood

木 The energy of Wood signifies dynamic movement and new beginnings. It is exemplified by the new shoots of spring, pushing vigorously through the ground after winter. Wood has an upward expansive energy, and this needs to harnessed if it is to be employed gainfully.

Sometimes Wood people direct their energy against themselves. Wood should be pliant and flexible; disharmonies produce a stiffness and hardness that give rise to aggression and violence. When in harmony, the energy of Wood is directed and deliberate, with a clear sense of vision. The eyes are the sense organ of the Liver, the organ relating to the Yin qualities of Wood, together with the Gall Bladder. If there is disharmony, the vision can be poor, both literally and in a much broader sense.

Wood energy is limited (the immature growth of spring must give way to the ripeness of summer), so the Wood type must always be aware of conserving energy.

RIGHT **Spring is synonymous with Wood, with a burst of energy stimulating new growth.**

RIGHT **Wood is allied to movement and the spring, when the growing season starts.**

Which Element are you? Wood

AFFINITIES
Liver and Gall Bladder, spring, sour tastes, tendons, eyes, the colour green, a shouting voice, wind and movement.

KEY WORDS
Movement, dynamism, organization, anger, frustration, rigidity, violence.

PRONE TO
Mood swings, depression, IBS, period problems, eye problems, gallstones, alcohol and substance abuse, insomnia with nightmares, violent behaviour.

KEY HERBS
Dang Gui, Bai Shao, Gou Qi Zi, Ju Hua, Chai Hu, Xiang Fu, Yu Jin.

RECOMMENDED FOODS
Green vegetables, oily fish, red and orange root vegetables, green tea, organic liver, olive oil, sesame oil.

FOODS TO AVOID
Alcohol, coffee (including decaffeinated), hot/spicy/greasy foods, caffeinated drinks, large amounts of pickles and vinegar.

CULTIVATE
• Relaxing activities such as meditation, gardening, painting, Tai Qi or yoga.

• A healthy relationship with your anger. Do not bottle up petty grievances and then explode inappropriately.

• A rhythmic exercise routine such as swimming or jogging.

ESSENTIALS
Wood people need to beware of over-activity, anger and over-exuberance.

Fire people make good leaders, but they can also be restless and hyperactive.

Fire

RIGHT **Fire is linked with the colour red, heat and the summer, when we can all enjoy being outdoors.**

Which Element are you? Fire

AFFINITIES
Heart and Small Intestine, summer, growth, bitter tastes, the complexion, tongue, speech, the colour red, a laughing voice, hot weather and hot conditions.

KEY WORDS
Happiness, love, excitement, joy, visionary, anxiety, indulgence, mania.

PRONE TO
Anxiety, over-stimulation, poor circulation, broken veins, bad complexion, restless sleep, dreaming, indecision, feeble memory, lack of communication skills, talking too much, hyperactivity.

KEY HERBS
Suan Zao Ren, Bai Zi Ren, Hou Ma Ren, Yuan Zhi, Ling Zhi, Dan Shen, Lian Zi, Huang Qin, Hong Hua.

RECOMMENDED FOODS
Oily fish; salads with bitter leaves such as endive, radicchio, dandelion; dates and longan fruit; herb teas made from leaves and flowers.

FOODS TO AVOID
Stimulants such as coffee and sugar, excessive spicy foods.

CULTIVATE
• A quiet pastime that will keep your feet on the ground, such as gardening.

• The qualities of leadership, empathy and compassion.

• An early bedtime.

火 Fire symbolizes the divine nature of human experience at its most fulfilled. Joy and happiness are found where there is light and warmth: fire penetrates the shadows and scatters the dark – the Fire Element is uplifting.

Fire Element people tend to be natural leaders who inspire the people around them, attracting loyalty and devotion. The Fire organ of the Heart is the centre of the emotions, and the Heart is said to be responsible for communication with others. Fire people are therefore able to articulate their feelings fully and are fond of talking.

The emotional aspects of the Heart are sensitive to external influences. Fire can burn too brightly or fade if it is not properly maintained. The need for social contact may also lead to mental overactivity. The Heart is said to house the Shen, our individual consciousness, and the Shen requires rest and tranquillity if it is to be maintained in harmony. It this does not happen, there will frequently be unease, anxiety and sleep problems.

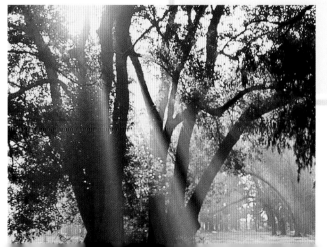

LEFT **Long, sun-dappled summer days reflect the happy nature of Fire.**

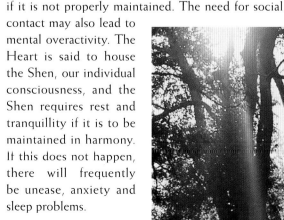

THE EIGHT CONDITIONS

Yin and Yang alone cannot adequately describe the complexity of human experience. To solve this problem, the Chinese devised the Eight Conditions, or Ba Gang. The Eight Conditions can be used to communicate any characteristic or disharmony, and are the main method used for categorizing people. By applying these principles to yourself, you will be able to identify your own particular strengths and weaknesses and avoid the imbalances that can lead to illness.

ABOVE **Yin and Yang – the tinted opposites – are one of the four pairs that make up the Eight Conditions.**

The four sets

The Eight Conditions are essentially interdependent characteristics, paired into four sets. This approach of using opposing, or bipolar, forces is in keeping with the Taoist philosophy of Yin and Yang. To be quite accurate, this system considers Yin and Yang to be 'superordinate' – they subsume and encompass the other three pairs. The four sets within the Eight Conditions are:

- Yin-Yang;
- Hot-Cold;
- Full-Empty; and
- Interior-Exterior.

These Eight Conditions can mix and match to cover the full range of disharmonies it is possible for people to develop. In complex patterns of disharmony, it is quite feasible for many of the Conditions to coexist in the same person, even apparently contradictory aspects such as Hot and Cold.

YIN-YANG

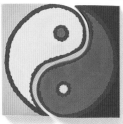

ABOVE **The attraction of opposites: interlocking and interdependent.**

We have already looked at the general concept of Yin-Yang. Depending on whether your personal characteristics tend towards either Yin or Yang, it is possible to gain an overview of your general body type. Which of the following descriptions fits you best?

YIN

YIN PEOPLE

Yin people are generally quiet and reserved, and tend to seek out a role at home or work where they can be supportive to others. They are careful and relaxed, and happy to enjoy a quiet life.

YIN ILLNESS

Chronic problems that develop over a period of time, and which drag on, are Yin illnesses. People with too much Yin need warming and drying, using herbs to strengthen Yang and Qi, and disperse Dampness.

YANG

YANG PEOPLE

Yang people are extrovert and outgoing, forceful and dynamic. They are hard to ignore! They tend to choose careers that allow them to display these abilities. They have lots of energy, do not feel the cold, and find it difficult to wind down and relax.

YANG ILLNESS

Sudden, acute symptoms (which are relatively severe) such as fever, swellings, thirst, and even convulsions, are typical Yang illnesses. There will often be Heat conditions and dramatic reactions. People with too much Yang need to be cooled and calmed, using herbs to nourish the Yin, detoxify and moisten the system, and calm the spirit.

ESSENTIALS
An imbalance or over-dominance of one characteristic leads to ill-health.

Knowing your body type can help you to prevent future health problems.

HOT-COLD

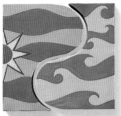

ABOVE **Hot and Cold. Heat is a Yang influence; Cold is related to Yin.**

A lot of disharmonies can be seen as either Hot or Cold. Yang people tend to get problems linked with Heat, whereas Yin people veer towards Cold symptoms.

HOT ILLNESSES

CHARACTERISTICS

Redness, feverishness, thirst, dryness, strong symptoms, sudden occurrence and activity, and often (but not invariably) in the upper part of the body. Pain is burning or acidic. If the patient comes into contact with warmth, this will worsen the problems, adding to the Heat already in the body. Heat turns Body Fluids dark yellow, or makes them green and thick.

EXAMPLES

Indigestion that comes on suddenly after too much alcohol, with burning pain rising upwards.

A typical sinus infection, with sudden pain and some thick yellow-green nasal discharge, inflammation and possibly a fever.

Anger, irritation, a quick temper, red face, severe headaches, a tendency to high blood-pressure.

COLD ILLNESSES

CHARACTERISTICS

Darkened areas, feelings of cold, increased fluids, slow onset, and lack of movement. Problems most often occur in the lower part of the body. Pain is cramping, twisting or tight in nature. Large amounts of white or clear Body Fluids.

EXAMPLES

A bladder chill: feelings of cold, backache, lack of thirst, and lots of clear urine.

Joint pain that worsens in cold weather, stiffness, and feelings of tiredness. Abdominal cramps and watery diarrhoea following too much cold food.

FULL-EMPTY

The Full-Empty set allows us to ascertain the relative strength or weakness of a disharmony, and that of the person suffering from it.

FULL CONDITIONS

CHARACTERISTICS

Severe symptoms denote Fullness. These will often

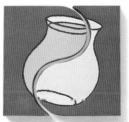

ABOVE **Full and Empty. Fullness reflects an excess, Emptiness reveals a lack.**

come on suddenly, flare up, and then die down quickly. Essentially, a Full condition is due to an over-abundance of something in the body.

SYMPTOMS

Sudden and severe pain, severe or pronounced mental agitation, acute conditions.

EXAMPLES

A common cold that develops rapidly with thick catarrh, sweating, raised temperature and a rasping sore throat, indicating an Excess of Heat.

EMPTY CONDITIONS

CHARACTERISTICS

A lack of something in the body. The disharmony usually develops quite slowly, is chronic in nature, and has relatively mild symptoms.

SYMPTOMS

Weakness, feebleness, dull pain, lethargy, sleepiness, and most chronic conditions.

EXAMPLES

Coldness in the body which feels better when heated.

INTERIOR-EXTERIOR

The last of the four sets refers to the area of the body in which the disharmony manifests itself.

EXTERIOR CONDITIONS

CHARACTERISTICS

Exterior conditions are those which affect the skin and muscles. In Chinese Medicine, this really refers

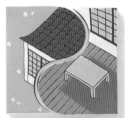

ABOVE **Interior and Exterior. These descriptions refer to the site of a problem.**

to colds, flu and viruses, where the first symptoms are aching muscles, fever, chilliness, a stiff neck or a rash. (However, not all skin diseases are classified as Exterior: most are due to an Interior condition that is manifesting in the skin. Only those skin rashes that are associated with an illness such as measles or chicken pox are classified as Exterior conditions.)

INTERIOR CONDITIONS

CHARACTERISTICS

Interior conditions are all those diseases that are not Exterior conditions. In Chinese Medicine this means that anything affecting the internal organs of the body – the Spleen, Lungs, Kidneys, Liver, Heart and so on – is considered to be an Interior problem. If minor Exterior problems are not treated, then they can move into the Interior of the body, where they may possibly become chronic or life-threatening.

Working out a pattern of disharmony

Once you understand the Eight Conditions, you will be able to use them to classify any problem you come across. Remember that any combination is possible, and that more than one condition may occur simultaneously. Looking at problems in this way becomes natural with practice.

FULL-HEAT

⚕ CHARACTERISTICS

As for Hot and Full patterns.

⚕ SYMPTOMS

Fever, high thirst, red face and red eyes, strong movements, feeling hot to the touch, burning pain, manic behaviour, darkening of Body Fluids, bright red tongue and fast pulse.

⚕ HERBS

Cooling and detoxifying herbs.

EMPTY-HEAT

⚕ CHARACTERISTICS

Heat symptoms resulting from a lack, or Deficiency, of Yin. This causes the Yin functions of cooling and moistening to become impaired, and leads to too much, or an Excess, of Yang Heat in the body.

⚕ SYMPTOMS

Typically, symptoms are chronic rather than acute, and less pronounced than for Full-Heat illnesses. So, there will be flushing rather than fever, a dry mouth instead of high thirst, general dryness, red cheeks, and anxiety or restlessness.

⚕ HERBS

Herbs that nourish the Yin are needed to counterbalance the over-active Yang energy that has built up in the body. These include moist herbs that strengthen the body's Fluids and Blood.

Susan's case

Susan wakes up one morning with a sudden urge to urinate. When she passes water, there is a strong burning sensation and the urine is dark yellow, concentrated, and has a strong smell. She starts to feel hot and goes to her doctor, who diagnoses cystitis. In Chinese Medicine, cystitis can be an Exterior condition caused by invading Evils – in this case an Excess of Heat. If the condition is untreated, it will start to affect the Interior and can then lead to an Internal Heat condition.

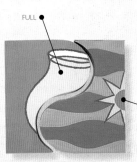

FULL

HOT

ABOVE **Susan has Heat, from burning urine. Her sudden, severe symptoms reflect Fullness.**

Helen's case

Helen's periods have been getting more irregular and erratic over the last couple of years, and her doctor says that she is going through the menopause. She gets hot flushes several times a day, and is finding she feels anxious in situations that previously would not have bothered her. Her sleep is restless. She notices that her skin and hair have become dry. Helen has Empty-Heat due to a lack of Yin, a natural occurrence in a woman who has had a lifetime of periods. According to Chinese theory, the Empty-Heat is believed to be invading the Heart, which is the seat of many emotions. This leads to the anxiety, restlessness and tearfulness commonly associated with menopausal upsets.

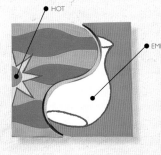

HOT

EMPTY

ABOVE **Helen has too much Heat. Her lack of Yin makes this an Empty condition.**

BAI HE

RIGHT **Bai He nourishes Yin, boosting the Heart and Lungs. It is good for Empty-Heat problems, such as Helen's symptoms.**

FULL-COLD

✿ CHARACTERISTICS

An excess of Cold, causing Stagnation and the slowing down of body functions.

✿ SYMPTOMS

Feeling cold and not being able to warm up, stiffness, cramping or twisting pain, a lack of thirst, a desire for warmth, and frequent copious urination. The skin can darken or go bluish-purple, the tongue may be dark or pale, and the pulse is slow.

✿ HERBS

As well as removing the source of the Cold by warming the body, heating herbs are used to warm the Yang and scatter the invading Cold.

EMPTY-COLD

✿ CHARACTERISTICS

Deficiency of Yang or Heat, leading to a relative Excess of the Yin cooling and moistening functions.

✿ SYMPTOMS

Feelings of cold, cold limbs (which feel better for the application of warmth), lack of thirst, aversion to cold, lethargy, diarrhoea (due to a weakness of the Digestive Fire), inability to hold water in the bladder for a long time, a feeble pulse and a pale tongue. Empty-Cold can be common in the elderly, weak or malnourished when there is a general run-down of the Yang. Certain Yang energies diminish naturally with age, which is why Empty-Cold is quite common.

✿ HERBS

Herbs are needed to strengthen the Qi and Yang, without damaging the Yin. Drying herbs are needed to clear the Excess Dampness, but it is important to regulate their use to prevent damage to bodily fluids, which would affect the Yin.

Owen's case

Owen has been out chopping wood for several hours. It is below freezing and he has some pain in his fingers, which is getting worse. He goes inside and tries to warm his hands by the fire, but they have gone purple and feel icy. Prompt action is required if frostbite is to be avoided. The intense Cold has invaded the peripheries of the body and needs to be treated quickly while it is still an Exterior issue, before it moves to the Interior and causes more damage.

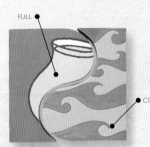

FULL

COLD

Eddie's case

Eddie has always had a weight problem, but over the last few years he has put on a lot of weight and feels tired all the time. His doctor runs tests and finds that his thyroid gland is underactive. Eddie's problem is due to a lack of Yang energy, so his Metabolic Fire is weak, resulting in weight gain and lethargy. Lack of Yang also contributes to his general feelings of tiredness, while the resulting Excess of Yin leads to an imbalance in the body's Fluids, leading to weight gain. Eddie feels cold because of the over-abundance of Yin.

COLD

EMPTY

ABOVE **Owen has subjected himself to freezing temperatures, which have caused an Excess of Cold.**

ABOVE **Eddie's underactive thyroid gland causes a Deficiency of Yang, and he feels the cold.**

ESSENTIALS
Any combination of the Eight Conditions may occur.

—

Consider all the symptoms carefully before diagnosing.

THE SEASONS AND YOUR HEALTH

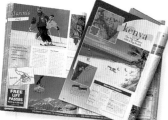

Modern life tends to prevent us from staying in touch with the seasons. It is entirely possible to ignore the main effects of the weather when we are cocooned by central heating, air conditioning and double glazing. However, no matter how much you protect yourself from the environment, your Qi is still tuned to the time of year.

ABOVE **The speed of modern travel enables us to flit easily between time zones, jumping from one season to another – but what effect will this have on our Qi?**

BAI SHAO FOR SPRING, A TONIC FOR THE BLOOD

SPRING

Seasonal affinities

Good health is maintained by harmonizing with the seasons. In spring it is appropriate to become more active after long winter months spent indoors; in summer we can relax and enjoy the warm weather; and in autumn we should start to gather together our resources for the winter.

There are five seasons according to the Chinese view: spring, summer, autumn, winter, and the transitional stage at the end of each season, when one season changes to another. Each season is linked with an Element, and shares the same characteristics; for example, summer and Fire are both related to growth, warmth, and joy. These qualities will also be possible weaknesses for a person with a dominance of the Element that relates to the season. For example the Water type (related to winter) may well be more susceptible to cold and dark weather than most people.

DANG SHEN IS THE APPROPRIATE HERB FOR ALL FOUR TRANSITIONAL STAGES, A TONIC FOR THE QI

WINTER

THE FIVE CLIMATES

The Five Climates refer to the environmental conditions that prevail in each of the four seasons, together with the transition period. The Five Climates are the natural type of weather for a particular season – hot in summer and cold in winter. When the weather is wrong for the time of year, as is increasingly the case as the effects of global climate change become apparent, then seasonal illness may result.

SHU DI HUANG FOR WINTER, TO NOURISH THE BLOOD

RIGHT **Living in harmony with the seasons helps to maintain healthy Qi. Herbs help to redress imbalances caused by weather conditions.**

DANG SHEN, A TONIC FOR THE QI

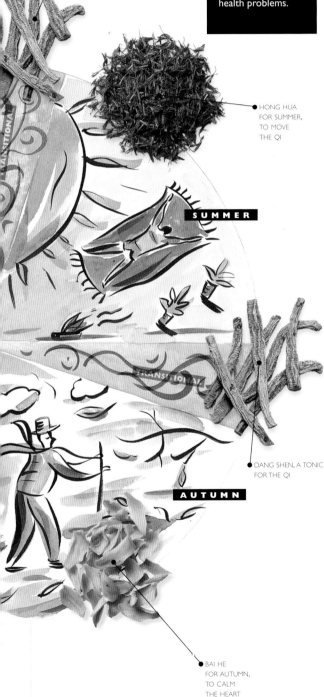

DANG SHEN, A
TONIC FOR THE QI

HONG HUA
FOR SUMMER,
TO MOVE
THE QI

TRANSITIONAL

SUMMER

TRANSITIONAL

DANG SHEN, A TONIC
FOR THE QI

AUTUMN

BAI HE
FOR AUTUMN,
TO CALM
THE HEART

SPRING

In springtime, the energy hibernating beneath the
earth bursts forth with the first warm rays of the sun.
This is a time of rapid change and development.

ELEMENT: **WOOD**

Spring is the time of Wind. The Chinese character
for Wind, or Feng, is a violent gust carrying a small
insect. This symbol conveys the idea of illness carried
through the air. Wind implies movement, usually
of a violent nature, or a lack of it. Spring is a time of
new beginnings, when energy and movement are vigorous and ascending. Wind also brings with it the
idea of change and new growth (we talk about the
'wind of change' in our own culture).

ADVICE FOR SPRING

Spring is thought to be the time when we are particularly susceptible to colds and viruses, and when
allergies are likely to start up. So, it is important to
protect yourself from the effects of Wind by dressing
warmly, and in particular, avoiding draughts on your
neck or chest. If you have a tendency to catch colds,
and especially if you are a Metal type, choose herbs
that will strengthen the Qi and Lungs to protect you.
If you suffer from hay fever, select herbs from the
Phlegm category; also Liver herbs, as Wind relates to
spring, the associated season of the Liver.

Take part in brisk activities. Eat less and more
simply, or engage in a detoxifying fast to clear the fats
stored up over winter. Eat light foods such as young
plants; also raw, sweet and pungent foods. Cook food
for a short time at a high temperature.

SUMMER

Summer sees growth come to fruition. We tend to
feel energized by the longer days and warmer nights,
and are full of the joys of life and love.

ELEMENT: **FIRE**

Summer is the time of Heat. Heat and Fire are Yang
energies. Yang is at its peak in the summer, expressed
through growth, brightness, activity, creativity
and joy. Heat is warming, drying, energizing and
activating. Heat is required for all transformative
processes to take place, for example cooking or the
growth of plants. Fire is a more destructive force – it
is Heat that has gone out of control.

The Heart, which is the organ relating to the Fire
Element, is particularly susceptible to the effects of
Heat. This can be seen in acute cases of heatstroke,
where the patient becomes incoherent and sweats

(the Heart controls speech and perspiration). In less acute situations, where Heat is due to the diet or emotions, the symptoms are similar but less extreme, for example insomnia or night sweats.

ADVICE FOR SUMMER

Fire Element people need to take care not to overheat, internally or externally, especially during the summer months. Choose herbs that calm the Mind if there is mental disturbance, and herbs to detoxify if there are signs of rampant Heat or Fire.

Eat colourful food, use spices, and cook food quickly. Use less salt and more water; drink warm liquids. Eat smaller, lighter meals on hot days.

SEASONAL TRANSITION

It is essential to match our behaviour and attitude to each new season, because the period of seasonal transition is when ill-health frequently occurs.

ELEMENT: **EARTH**

This is the period at the end of each season. It is a time to attune yourself to the season to come. Like Yin-Yang, the change from one season to another is a process, not a sudden event. This time of change relates to the transformative properties of the Earth Element. All things must return to the earth before they can be transformed into something else, and this applies to the seasons as well. Earth is the axis around which the seasons revolve.

ADVICE FOR SEASONAL TRANSITION

Eat simply. Earth Element types need to pay particular attention to their digestive systems. Regular meals, eaten slowly and when relaxed, are important. Choose foods such as sweet grains and vegetables. Prepare them plainly, with little seasoning, and eat only a few foods at each meal.

AUTUMN

Autumn brings clarity and simplicity. It is a time to prepare for the relative hibernation of winter.

ELEMENT: **METAL**

Autumn is the time of Dryness, when energy starts to move inwards and downwards, returning to the earth.

Like leaves, our skin may become drier. The Lungs and Large Intestine, which are the organs relating to Metal, can be injured by Dryness. The Lungs are susceptible if the central heating is turned on too early without the use of humidifiers, or if they are exposed to air-conditioning. If the Lungs are injured by

Dryness, constipation or a cough may result. Some types of asthma are exacerbated at this time of year.

ADVICE FOR AUTUMN

People who are susceptible to Dryness should choose herbs to strengthen the Qi and Lungs, or herbs which are moistening to the Lungs and both Intestines.

Prepare foods carefully to consolidate their energy. Focus on stimulating the sense of smell. Bake and sauté foods, and cook with less water on a low heat for longer. Gradually introduce sour, salty and bitter foods.

WINTER

In winter the long, dark nights push us into spending more time indoors, encouraging reflection and introspection. We are therefore less active.

ELEMENT: **WATER**

Winter is the time of Cold. Water is the Element that relates to winter, and the main action of Water is to cool and moisten. Water always sinks to the lowest level, where it will either nourish (as in feeding roots) or cause a blockage (if there is no circulation). Water requires movement to activate its functions, otherwise it will be Stagnant. In winter, energy travels deep into our bodies where it lies dormant until the spring. Therefore, the nature of Water is Cold.

The circulation of Qi and Blood are reduced by the effects of Cold. The contracting nature of Cold also stiffens the muscles and tendons and causes pain, especially in the back or knees. Water is linked to the Kidneys and Bladder, which play a major role in Water metabolism. Cold tends to increase the need to urinate, or causes water retention in the body.

ADVICE FOR WINTER

People with Cold present in the body, or who are very sensitive to cold, should choose herbs to strengthen the Yang and Qi, as well as herbs that move the Qi and Blood (if there is pain).

Keep warm, rest, meditate and conserve energy. Eat warming and hearty foods. Steam vegetables. Cook for longer, with less water, at a lower temperature. Use more sea salt, include bitter foods in your diet, and eat preserved and fermented foods such as miso (fermented soy bean paste).

The Five Flavours

Each Element has a particular flavour associated with it, and people will often get a craving for a taste when they have an imbalance – sweet cravings will frequently be experienced by people with a weak Earth energy. A small amount of the natural flavour for each Element will stimulate and strengthen the organ system connected to it. Try to eat foods from each taste category on a regular basis, aiming to find natural sources for each type.

Each flavour has an associated direction that refers to the nature of its Qi. Alcohol and spicy foods, for example, have an upwards and outwards energy. This means that they take the Qi in that direction, which is why you may feel flushed and perspire after consuming them. Lemon juice, on the other hand, is sour and has an inwards, astringent energy. This means that it will tend to close things off, so it can be used to treat loss of fluids, such as sweating or diarrhoea.

SWEET | EARTH

Sweetness has a Yang energy, can be cooling or warming, has an affinity with transition and change, moves upwards and outwards, tonifies, harmonizes, moistens Dryness (good), produces Dampness (bad), builds tissue (good), creates fat (bad).
Examples of sweet foods: carrot, pumpkin, parsnip, fruit, honey.

SALTY | WATER

Saltiness has a Yin energy, is cooling, has an affinity with the season of winter, moves downwards and inwards, regulates fluids, detoxifies, enters the Kidneys, softens (good), hardens (bad).
Examples of salty foods: seaweed, celery, shellfish, soy sauce.

BITTER | FIRE

Bitterness has a Yin energy, is cooling, has an affinity with summer, has a descending movement, reduces Excess, promotes digestion, dries Dampness (good), causes Dryness (bad).
Examples of bitter foods: radicchio, rye, rhubarb, coffee.

SOUR | WOOD

Sourness has a Yin energy, is cooling, has an affinity with spring, is contracting and astringent, stops leakage, consolidates (good), makes tense (bad).
Examples of sour foods: grapefruit, trout, tomato.

PUNGENT | METAL

Pungency has a Yang energy, is warming, has an affinity with autumn, moves upwards and outwards, promotes circulation, aids digestion, induces sweating, distributes (good), scatters (bad).
Examples of pungent foods: ginger, onion, cabbage.

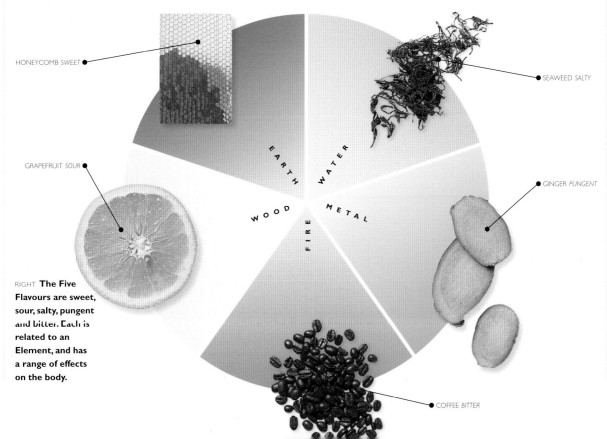

HONEYCOMB *SWEET*

SEAWEED *SALTY*

GRAPEFRUIT *SOUR*

GINGER *PUNGENT*

E A R T H

W A T E R

W O O D

M E T A L

F I R E

RIGHT **The Five Flavours are sweet, sour, salty, pungent and bitter. Each is related to an Element, and has a range of effects on the body.**

COFFEE *BITTER*

THE TWELVE ORGANS

The twelve organs are the Heart, Pericardium, Small Intestine, Triple Heater (San Jiao), Spleen, Stomach, Lungs, Large Intestine, Kidneys, Bladder, Liver and Gall Bladder. Each organ is Yin or Yang, and has an associated Element. The twelve main Channels, or Meridians, correspond to the twelve organs. The organs all have special roles to play.

The organs and their Elements

Each of the twelve organs is affiliated to one of the Five Elements, and assumes its characteristics. Each organ is either Yin or Yang; Yin organs have a corresponding Yang organ, and vice versa.

ELEMENT: **EARTH**

Yin organ: ● Spleen

Yang organ: ● Stomach

ELEMENT: **METAL**

Yin organ: ◆ Lungs

Yang organ: ● Large Intestine

ELEMENT: **WATER**

Yin organ: ≡ Kidneys

Yang organ: ▲ Bladder

ELEMENT: **WOOD**

Yin organ: ‖ Liver

Yang organ: ⎮ Gall Bladder

ELEMENT: **FIRE**

Yin organs: ◤ Heart

◢ Pericardium (Xin Bao)

Yang organs: ■ Small Intestine

▥ Triple Heater (San Jiao)

RIGHT **Each of the twelve Meridians (energy Channels) in the body corresponds to one of the twelve organs. There are three paired Yin Meridians and three paired Yang Meridians in the arm; likewise in the leg. The Yin Meridians are on the inside of the limb, the Yang Meridians are on the outside.**

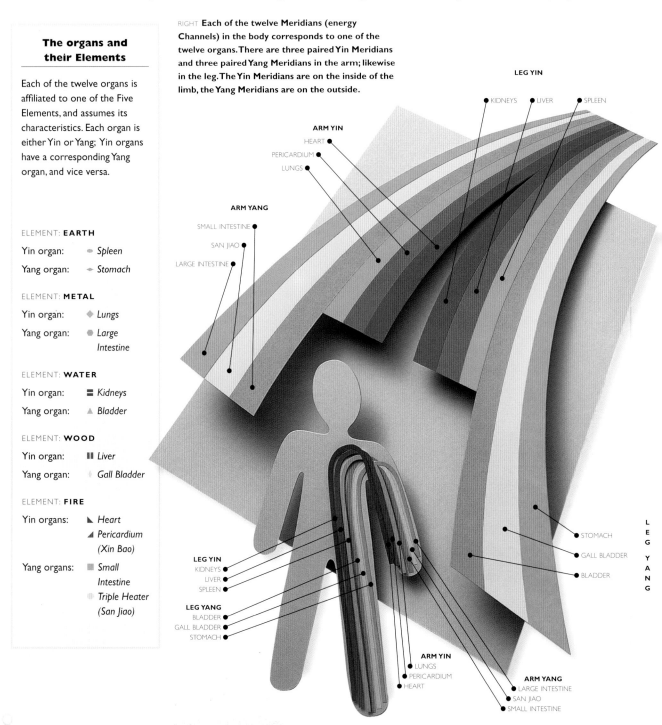

LEG YIN
KIDNEYS LIVER SPLEEN

ARM YIN
HEART
PERICARDIUM
LUNGS

ARM YANG
SMALL INTESTINE
SAN JIAO
LARGE INTESTINE

LEG YIN
KIDNEYS
LIVER
SPLEEN

LEG YANG
BLADDER
GALL BLADDER
STOMACH

ARM YIN
LUNGS
PERICARDIUM
HEART

STOMACH
GALL BLADDER
BLADDER

L E G   Y A N G

ARM YANG
LARGE INTESTINE
SAN JIAO
SMALL INTESTINE

Functions of the internal organs

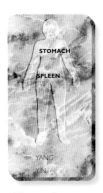

SPLEEN, STOMACH
The Spleen and Stomach are responsible for digestion, assimilation and distribution of nutrients and Water through the body. Their efficient function is vital for the upkeep of good health.

ELEMENT: Earth.

SUSCEPTIBILITY: Dampness.

EMOTIONAL ASPECTS: Tendency to worry, prone to brooding and pensiveness, may suffer from obsessive-compulsive disorders and vexation.

Main functions	Symptoms of disharmony
Governs digestion: Nutrients are extracted from food by the combined efforts of the Spleen and Stomach.	Bloating, poor appetite, tiredness, loose stools, weight gain, food intolerance, nausea, high or low thirst.
Raises the Pure upwards: The nutrients, also known as the Pure, rise up to the Heart and Lungs, where they are circulated by respiration.	Prolapse, diarrhoea, downward bleeding, spontaneous bruising.
Controls the limbs and muscles: Because the Spleen is so closely linked with nutrition, it controls the healthy development of limbs and muscles.	Heaviness and weakness of arms and legs. Poor muscle tone, atrophy, weakness.
Controls the mouth: The mouth and Spleen are related through the muscles, therefore the health of the Spleen is reflected in the lips.	Problems with sense of taste.
Houses the intellect: Intellect resides in the Spleen. Poor Spleen energy can cause mental confusion and forgetfulness.	Poor concentration and memory, muzzy-headedness.

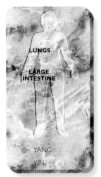

LUNGS, LARGE INTESTINE
The Lungs are responsible for respiration, controlling the flow of air and also the flow of Qi. They are linked to the Large Intestine, which expels solid waste from the body.

ELEMENT: Metal.

SUSCEPTIBILITY: Dryness, Phlegm and Cold.

EMOTIONAL ASPECTS: Grief, sadness.

Main functions	Symptoms of disharmony
Governs respiration: The Lungs are responsible for breathing, but also control the flow of Qi, dispersing the Wei Qi (defence energy) through the body and to the skin and muscles.	Weak voice, shortness of breath, tiredness, cold hands.
Controls the pores: In sending the Wei Qi to the skin, the Lungs also influence the pores.	Catching colds easily, spontaneous sweating, airborne allergies.
Controls the nose: Since air passes through the nose to the Lungs, the Chinese believe that the two organs are linked.	Poor sense of smell, sneezing, sinus problems.
Regulates the bowels: The action of breathing massages the colon via the diaphragm and helps to ensure regular bowel movements.	Constipation.

ESSENTIALS
The Zang (solid) organs are: Lungs, Spleen, Heart, Liver, Kidneys. The Fu (hollow) organs are: Bladder, Large and Small Intestines, Gall Bladder, Stomach and San Jiao.

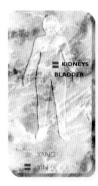

KIDNEYS, BLADDER

The Kidneys encourage growth and play a part in reproduction. They regulate Water and are associated with the Bladder.

ELEMENT: Water.

SUSCEPTIBILITY: Dryness, Cold.

EMOTIONAL ASPECTS: Fear, lack of will and motivation.

HOUSES THE GATE OF LIFE: The root of Qi.

Main functions	Symptoms of disharmony
Governs development and growth: The Kidneys store reproductive Qi, which is linked to inherited Qi.	Infertility, impotence, retarded development, premature ageing, menarche to menopause.
Produces bones and marrow: Marrow nurtures bones, assists brain function.	Weak bones and teeth, mental retardation, dizziness, low intelligence.
Governs Water: The Kidneys play a central role in controlling Body Fluids.	Profuse pale urination, scanty dark urination, the need to urinate at night, incontinence, cystitis, stones.
Controls the ears: Via the Meridians, the Kidneys are linked to the ears.	Deafness, impaired hearing, tinnitus.
Manifests in the head hair: Through Blood, hair is nourished by Kidney Jing.	Premature balding and greying.

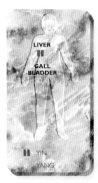

LIVER, GALL BLADDER

The Chinese credit the Liver with many more properties than the Western view of it as the body's chemical factory: it controls the Blood and Qi.

ELEMENT: Wood.

SUSCEPTIBILITY: Heat, Damp-Heat, Dryness.

EMOTIONAL ASPECTS: Anger, frustration, irritability, PMT.

Main functions	Symptoms of disharmony
Controls movement of Qi: Liver Qi is related to digestive function. Smoothly flowing Qi regulates emotions.	Stagnation of Qi, migraine, depression.
Stores the Blood: The Liver regulates the volume of Blood in the body. It is closely linked to menstruation, the eyes, tendons and sinews, and nails. The nails reflect the health of the Liver.	Irregular /painful /no /heavy periods, Stagnation of Blood. Poor vision, dry /gritty /bloodshot eyes, floaters, photophobia. Spasms, cramps, stiffness, tremors, tics. Nails dry, cracked, indented, dark or pale.
Secretes bile: The Gall Bladder is a bile reservoir, which aids digestion.	Stones, hypochondriac distension.

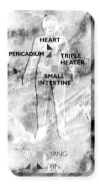

HEART, SMALL INTESTINE

The Heart rules the organs, controls life processes, and co-ordinates the action of the other Zang-Fu organs. The Small Intestine separates Pure from Impure after digestion.

ELEMENT: Fire.

SUSCEPTIBILITY: Heat.

EMOTIONAL ASPECTS: Over-enthusiasm, inappropriate behaviour, mania.

HOUSES THE SHEN: The soul.

Main functions	Symptoms of disharmony
Governs the Blood: The Heart's Qi affects the vigour of blood flow.	Cold hands, lack of vigour, tiredness.
Manifests in the complexion: The many facial blood vessels can indicate the condition of the Heart (e.g. abundant Heart Heat gives a red complexion).	Cold: bright white. Heat: red. Blood Stagnation: blue-purple.
Houses the Spirit: The Heart is closely linked with emotions and mental activities, and also with the Shen, or Spirit.	Depression, anxiety, poor memory, insomnia, palpitations, indecision. Circulation problems, thread veins.
Controls the tongue: The Chinese traditionally associate the tongue with the Heart and speech.	Aphasia, stuttering, incessant talking, inappropriate laughter, poor communication.

The twelve officials

The *Nei Jing Su Wen* is a classic text written by Huang Di, the Yellow Emperor (2696–2598 BC). It is usually known in English as his *Classic of Internal Medicine.* Huang Di asked his physician, Qi Bo, to tell him about the twelve organs and their relationships. Qi Bo described them as twelve officials and government departments, adding that they must work in harmony to achieve good health.

ESSENTIALS
Each organ has functions, strengths, weaknesses and interdependencies.

The health of the organs is reflected in the body – such as pink lips showing a healthy Spleen.

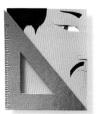
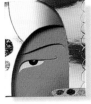

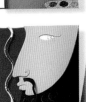

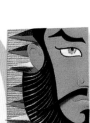
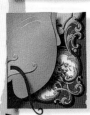
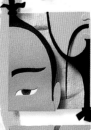

LUNGS
PRIME MINISTER
*Responsibility:
control and
regulation.*

HEART
THE EMPEROR
*Responsibility: the
brightness of the
Shen (Spirit-Mind).*

LIVER
GENERAL OF THE
EMPEROR'S ARMIES
*Responsibility:
planning and
deliberation.*

**PERICARDIUM
(XIN BAO)**
OFFICE OF THE
ENVOYS AND
AMBASSADORS
*Responsibility: joy
and happiness.*

GALL BLADDER
OFFICE OF CORRECT
ORIENTATION
*Responsibility:
decisiveness*

KIDNEYS
OFFICE FOR ACTIVATION OF
POWER AND STRENGTH
*Responsibility: special
skills and adeptness.*

LARGE INTESTINE
OFFICE OF
COMMUNICATION ROUTES
*Responsibility:
transformation
and change.*

**SPLEEN AND
STOMACH**
OFFICE OF GRANARIES
AND STOREHOUSES
*Responsibility:
the Five Flavours.*

**TRIPLE HEATER
(SAN JIAO)**
OFFICE FOR CONSTRUCTION
OF CHANNELS
Responsibility: Water pathways.

BLADDER
OFFICE OF THE
REGIONAL CAPITALS
*Responsibility: Fluid storage
and transformation.*

SMALL INTESTINE
OFFICE FOR
RECEPTION OF PLENTY
*Responsibility: transformed
substances.*

DAMP, PHLEGM AND FOOD STAGNATION

Our eating habits may cause the digestion to function poorly, leaving behind residues known as Damp, Phlegm or Stagnant Food. The Western diet is particularly likely to cause the formation of these residues, and many of the medical and dietary conditions that are on the increase today can be related to their effects: food sensitivities and intolerance, chronic candidiasis, ME and asthma.

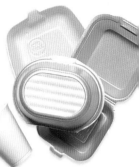

ABOVE **Junk foods contribute to Damp, Phlegm and Food Stagnation.**

The causes

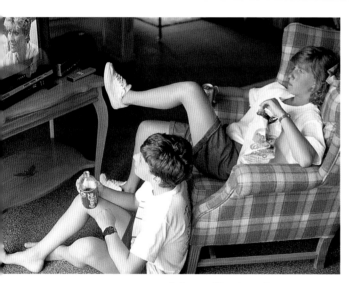

ABOVE **Sedentary lifestyles and poor nutrition contribute to dietary problems in the West.**

Various factors, such as a history of dieting, contribute to Dampness, Phlegm and Food Stagnation. The way we eat, too, has an influence: habits such as overfilling the stomach, incomplete chewing, eating too fast, and drinking too much cold fluid with food. Certain foods are especially likely to cause residues: an excess of sweet, raw or sticky food; dairy produce, including eggs; wheat, yeast, and to a lesser extent rye, corn and millet; animal fats, iced food or drinks, excessive alcohol, processed or artificially preserved foods.

DAMP

Normal Body Fluids (Jin Ye) have the function of moistening and lubricating the skin, mucous membranes, synovial tissues, etc. If Body Fluids coagulate or become thick, they become pathological and are known as Damp. Dampness will commonly combine with an existing influence in the body to become Damp-Heat or Damp-Cold.

CHARACTERISTICS OF DAMP

- It is heavy and tends to sink downwards.
- It impedes the function of the organs.
- It impedes the flow of Qi and Blood.
- It can be observed in the body excretions.
- It can be observed on the tongue.

SITES OF DISHARMONY

Spleen, Large Intestine, Bladder.

Organ	Common Damp problem
Spleen	Little appetite, bloating, loose stools, tiredness, lethargy, heaviness of the body and limbs, poor mental function, food intolerance.
Large Intestine	Diarrhoea, mucus in the stools, sticky bowel movements with tenesmus (straining), incomplete bowel movements.
Bladder	Cystitis.

RIGHT **Conventional anatomy, as taught to Western doctors. The Chinese concept of the body organs credits them with many functions unrecognized by Western medicine.**

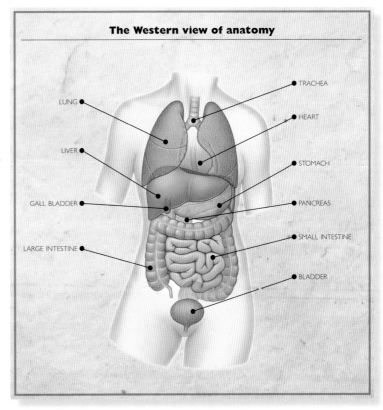

The Western view of anatomy

TRACHEA
HEART
LUNG
STOMACH
LIVER
PANCREAS
GALL BLADDER
SMALL INTESTINE
LARGE INTESTINE
BLADDER

DAMP-HEAT

The combination of Dampness and Heat is very commonly seen in the West. Dampness which sits around and Stagnates will generate Heat, rather like a compost heap. Damp-Heat is a poison. It is the most commonly seen element in diseases such as AIDS, myalgic encephalomyelitis (ME or chronic fatigue syndrome) and cancer. Damp-Heat is also associated with with red skin eruptions, such as blisters, cold sores and shingles.

CHARACTERISTICS

Swellings, itching, suppuration, oozing, foul and yellow discharges, infections, jaundice, inflammations. Any weeping sore, abscess, or ulcer generally indicates a degree of Damp-Heat syndrome. It is commonly present in post-viral fatigue syndrome.

SITES OF DISHARMONY

Liver, Gall Bladder, Spleen, Stomach, Large Intestine, Bladder, and Lower Jiao.

FOODS THAT FORM DAMP-HEAT

Spicy and oily food such as curries; fried and greasy foods; sugars and sweets; tropical fruits and juices; coffee; alcohol.

Organ	Common Damp-Heat problem
Liver	Jaundice, sclerosis, some skin conditions, shingles.
Gall Bladder	Stones, inflammation.
Lower Jiao	Genital infections, thrush, cystitis, prostatitis.
Stomach	Ulcers, indigestion.
Large Intestine	Colitis, dysentery.

DAMP-COLD

When Dampness and Cold both exist in the body, Damp-Cold is the result. This usually involves constriction of the circulation, stiffness and soreness in muscles and joints, tiredness and an aversion to cold. In the Bladder it can cause irritation of the urethra.

CHARACTERISTICS

As for Cold and Damp.

SITES OF DISHARMONY

Spleen, Bladder, Stomach.

FOODS THAT PROMOTE DAMP-COLD

Ice-cream, bananas, avocados, cold drinks, raw food.

Organ	Common Damp-Cold problem
Spleen	Poor appetite, tiredness, heaviness of the body; muscular aches and pains.
Bladder	Irritation of the urethra leading to frequent passing of cloudy urine, a tendency to urinary stones, and low backache.
Stomach	Nausea, vomiting, lack of thirst, abdominal cramping pains and watery diarrhoea.

PHLEGM

Mucus has the function of moistening the lungs and nose. Pathological mucus is called Phlegm. This is the phlegm or catarrh you see when it is coughed up. It is formed from Stagnant Damp and from the action of Heat or Cold on normal mucus.

CHARACTERISTICS
✿ Phlegm: made by the Spleen, housed in the Lungs.
✿ Strange diseases are caused by Phlegm.
✿ Asthma always involves Phlegm.

SITES OF DISHARMONY
Phlegm tends to be in the middle to upper body, either in the Lungs or Stomach. It is also seen in lumps under the skin, such as ganglia, lymphomas, lypomas (fatty lumps under the skin), some tumours, some ovarian cysts and an enlarged thyroid.

PHLEGM-HEAT

As with Dampness, Phlegm is most commonly associated with another existing influence on the body. Phlegm-Heat syndromes generally involve production of thick, yellow sputum with fever, dry mouth, lips and stools. The tongue is usually coated with a yellow film and the patient is irritable and restless.

CHARACTERISTICS
Phlegm-Heat is produced when there is too much Heat in the Lungs or Stomach. This can be caused by smoking tobacco, or by anxiety.

SITES OF DISHARMONY
Lungs, Stomach.

FOODS THAT FORM PHLEGM-HEAT
Alcohol, spicy food.

Organ	Common Phlegm-Heat problem
Lungs	Smoking-related problems, acute viral infections, allergic rhinitis, asthma. Yellow-green mucus, possibly blood-streaked, and either copious or hard to expectorate, depending on the level of Dryness of the Lungs.
Stomach	Thirst, hunger (but difficulty eating), acidity. Neurosis, severe delusional states, and psychiatric illness.

PHLEGM-COLD

The sputum is likely to be thin and foamy; the patient feels cold and complains of painful joints and stiffness. The tongue will have a white, moist coating.

CHARACTERISTICS
Phlegm-Cold is produced when the Lungs or Spleen are too Cold. This is often seen in children, the obese, and people who tend to catch colds easily. Phlegm-Cold can easily turn to Phlegm-Heat in an acute disease.

SITES OF DISHARMONY
Lungs, Spleen, Stomach.

Organ	Common Phlegm-Cold problem
Lungs	Irritating coughs and chest problems. The mucus is white and sticky, copious and easily expectorated. Possibly shortness of breath.
Spleen	Digestive upsets with abdominal bloating, poor appetite and discomfort.
Stomach	Distress caused by eating cold food and liquids, dairy foods, too much worry. Reduced appetite, nausea, vomiting, anorexia, dizziness, hypertension.

PHLEGM IN THE TISSUES

This refers to symptoms that are attributable to Phlegm, but where the Phlegm cannot be seen. It is often found in cases of a psychological nature. This type of Phlegm is said to 'cloud the Mind' and when the Mind is blocked, stroke, coma and epilepsy (Wind-Phlegm) may occur.

It is often involved in circulatory obstruction such as paralysis, multiple sclerosis, arterial sclerosis and coronary artery disease; also Parkinson's disease, Alzheimer's disease and Huntingdon's disease.

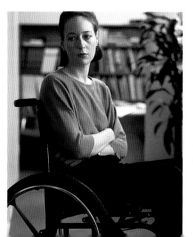

RIGHT **The Chinese regard Phlegm as a contributory factor to multiple sclerosis.**

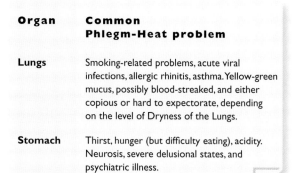

Stagnant Food

If the Stomach is crammed full, a large meal is eaten too late at night, or heavy or greasy food is consumed, then Food Stagnation may result. This pattern is the most commonly seen disharmony in children, where it is often referred to as Accumulation Syndrome.

CHILDREN

Infants have an inherently weak and immature digestion, and modern feeding habits (such as demand-feeding, bottle-feeding of formula or cow's milk, solid food too early) tend to exacerbate this. Many children eat a staple diet of fruit juice, bananas, yoghurts, sweets and crisps. These all lead to the formation of Stagnant Food, which in turn produces Dampness and Phlegm. If we look at the most common paediatric

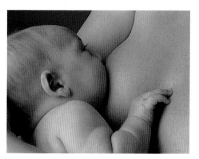

ABOVE **Breastfeeding is best; bottle-feeding may cause digestive upsets.**

LEFT **As children get older, add simple, nutritious foods to their diet.**

disorders (asthma, colic, fever, runny nose, glue ear, coughs, hyperactivity, and crying at night) we will start to see a connection between diet and health.

An infant's diet, up to nine months, should consist of milk (if not breastfeeding, use sheep's milk, which is closer than cow's to human milk; sterilize and store in the fridge). Between twelve and eighteen months, introduce rice porridge made with water. By the age of three, steamed or boiled vegetables and fruit should be given Broths made from lean meat or fish can be eaten if the child is of a poor constitution.

ADULTS

In adults it is possible to see either acute or chronic Food Stagnation. An acute pattern is usually due to overeating, resulting in an uncomfortable feeling in the stomach or bloating, which is not relieved until the food is digested or vomiting has taken place.

Chronic Food Stagnation occurs in those who overeat, have a bad diet, or diet excessively. It is usually part of a pattern of Dampness or Phlegm, and is a contributory factor in many food sensitivities.

General herbs for Dampness, Phlegm and Food Stagnation

REN SHEN

HERBS TO STRENGTHEN THE QI
The Spleen is the main Damp-producing organ, so herbs that strengthen the Qi of the Spleen and Stomach are good.

HERBS: *Ren Shen, Huang Qi, Shan Yao, Bai Zhu, Dang Shen, Zhi Gan Cao.*

YI ZHI REN

HERBS TO STRENGTHEN THE YANG
Some of these herbs have a warming action on the Spleen, assisting in the transformation of Dampness.

HERBS: *Yi Zhi Ren, Sheng Jiang, Hu Jiao, Rou Dou Kou.*

CHEN PI

HERBS TO AID THE DIGESTION
To some extent there must be a weakness of the digestion for Dampness to form; these herbs augment the action of the other herbs.

HERBS: *Chen Pi, Shan Zha, Mai Ya, Gu Ya, Shen Qu.*

HAI ZAO

HERBS TO COOL AND TRANSFORM HOT PHLEGM AND DAMPNESS
To clear Hot and Dry Phlegm and Dampness causing coughs and skin disorders.

HERBS: *Ze Xie, Bei Mu, Fu Ling, Yi Yi Ren, Qian Hu, Gua Lou, Tian Hua Fen, Zhu Li, Zhu Ru, Kun Bu, Hai Zao.*

LIAN QIAO

HERBS TO TRANSFORM COLD PHLEGM AND DAMPNESS
These herbs are warming.

HERBS: *Ban Xia, Tian Nan Xing, Bai Fu Zi, Xuan Fu Hua, Bai Qian, Bai Jie Zi, Jie Geng, Zao Jiao, Huo Xiang, Xing Ren, Cang Zhu, Sha Ren.*

JIN YIN HUA

HERBS TO CLEAR HEAT AND DETOXIFY
If there is Damp-Heat or Phlegm-Heat, it is appropriate to use herbs from this category.

HERBS: *Jin Yin Hua, Lian Qiao, Ju Hua, Pu Gong Yin, Cang Er Zi, Huang Lian, Huang Qin, Huang Bai.*

THE DIAGNOSTIC TOOLBOX

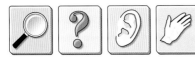

ABOVE **The Four Methods of diagnosis: looking, asking, listening and palpation.**

In Chinese Medicine, diagnosis is a very different process to that of Western medicine. The Chinese developed an almost poetical or euphemistic way of describing anatomy and physiology. In keeping with the whole of Taoist thinking, the internal workings of the body were likened to phenomena seen in the natural world. Therefore, much of Chinese Medicine is described in terms such as rivers, seas, fire, earth and wood. Early Chinese physicians had to depend on what they could see or feel as any sort of anatomical study or dissection was not widely practised.

ABOVE **A Chinese physician will examine a problem area by palpation.**

The tongue

A Chinese diagnosis involves Four Methods: looking, asking, listening and palpation. **Looking** is the observation of the tongue, hands, face, nails, skin, the patient's body type, and the way the patient moves.

Asking is when information about the existing condition and previous medical history is acquired.

Listening includes listening to the response to questions, but also means taking note of the tone of voice, breathing, body sounds, etc.

Palpation mainly involves taking the pulse, but may also include body palpation if appropriate.

OBSERVING THE TONGUE

The tongue is a major diagnostic tool. It is considered to be the only internal organ that can be seen from the outside, so, for a Chinese physician, looking at the tongue is like seeing an X-ray or a magnetic resonance imaging (MRI) scan of a patient.

The tongue provides an astonishing amount of information, both about existing illness and past and future health. By carefully observing your own tongue over a period of time, you can monitor your health and decide on the action required to cure illness, or as a preventative measure.

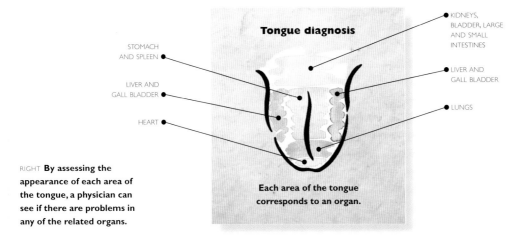

Tongue diagnosis

STOMACH AND SPLEEN

LIVER AND GALL BLADDER

HEART

KIDNEYS, BLADDER, LARGE AND SMALL INTESTINES

LIVER AND GALL BLADDER

LUNGS

Each area of the tongue corresponds to an organ.

RIGHT **By assessing the appearance of each area of the tongue, a physician can see if there are problems in any of the related organs.**

WHAT TO LOOK FOR

When looking at the tongue for diagnostic purposes, there are four things to take into consideration:

- Tongue colour.
- Tongue shape.
- Tongue coating.
- Distribution of cracks or spots.

It will often be necessary to cross-reference several or all of these aspects to establish a full picture. It is, of course, difficult to judge what is abnormal unless you know what a normal tongue looks like. A child's tongue can usually be regarded as a normal tongue: it should be fresh pink, have an even and symmetrical shape, have no cracks or spots, and should be topped with a thin coating of moisture.

Obviously every tongue is different, but there are a number of clear abnormalities which can help to pinpoint an imbalance; you will learn to recognize these with practice. The colour can range from the palest pink to bluish tints, while changes to the normal shape include unusual thinness, swellings, indentations or apparent tooth marks along one side.

The coating is especially important as the relative moistness or dryness of the tongue can be a good indicator of Yin or Yang dominance. The coating can also reveal the presence of Phlegm or Dampness. Monitoring changes in the tongue's appearance over time is more effective than trying to judge your health from an occasional quick look.

How to look at your tongue

- Observe your tongue in natural daylight to get a true picture of the colour and the coating.

- Open your mouth wide and stick the tongue out fully, but without straining. If the tongue is not relaxed, it will change the natural shape and colour.

- Don't rush the examination; it takes time to study the whole tongue. Note the position of any spots or blemishes.

- Recent food, drinks, vitamins or medicines can change the colour of the coating, so wait at least an hour after taking any of these before inspection.

- Looking at your tongue first thing in the morning, before you have brushed your teeth, reveals the coating in its full glory.

- Smoking and drinking tea may well produce marked changes in the quality of the coating.

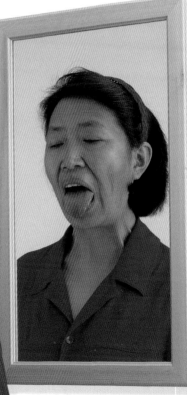

ABOVE **Check your tongue first thing in the morning and assess its colour, shape and coating; also see whether there are any cracks or spots.**

TONGUE COLOUR

Tongues come in many colours (some of which may sound surprising to you) depending on their state of health: pink, red, red-purple, blue-purple and blue.

PALE TONGUE

This can range from a slightly paler colour than normal, to almost white. A pale tongue is lighter than the fresh pink of a normal tongue. Generally, a pale tongue indicates a Deficiency. This might be a Deficiency of Qi, Yang or Blood.

RED TONGUE

This signifies Heat. The area of the redness indicates where the Heat is located in the body, and the depth of the redness shows how much Heat is present. The deeper the red, the more advanced the Heat condition. Additionally, the presence or absence of a tongue coating tells us if the Heat is due to a Full-Heat condition (Yang Excess), or an Empty-Heat condition (Yin Deficiency).

RED-PURPLE TONGUE

This is a stage further on from the red tongue. Purple indicates Stagnation of the Blood, usually resulting from Heat damage to the Blood.

BLUE-PURPLE TONGUE

This is a stage further on from a pale tongue. Purple indicates Stagnation of Blood, usually due to Cold from a Deficiency of something.

BLUE TONGUE

This is a tricky tongue to recognize. In an acute disease or a life-threatening emergency, the tongue may become blue due to a lack of oxygen, but in chronic illness the tongue may have a slight blue tinge. This indicates long-standing Cold in the body, which has damaged the Yang energy.

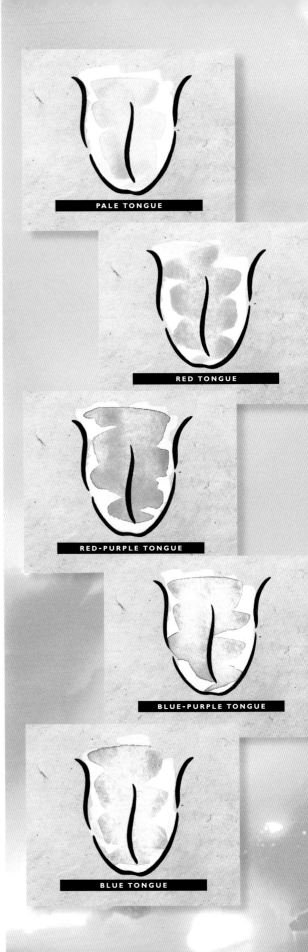

RIGHT **The colour of a tongue can vary from light pink to darker shades of red, sometimes verging towards blue. A pale tongue generally suggests some sort of Deficiency in the body, while a red tongue implies Heat – like an erupting volcano. Blue tints indicate Stagnation and the presence of Cold.**

PALE TONGUE

RED TONGUE

RED-PURPLE TONGUE

BLUE-PURPLE TONGUE

BLUE TONGUE

SWOLLEN TONGUE

THIN TONGUE

SWELLING IN ONE AREA

INDENTATION IN ONE AREA

LONG TONGUE

TONGUE SHAPE

A tongue can be long or short, and thin or swollen.
Specific areas may be indented or swollen.

SWOLLEN TONGUE

Swelling usually denotes a Deficiency of either Qi or
Yang, or the presence of Heat. A Yang or Qi
Deficiency will cause a pale, swollen tongue. If the
tongue is normal or red-coloured, it indicates Heat.

A rolled appearance to the sides of a swollen
tongue can show one of two things. Symptoms such
as loose stools, tiredness and bloating reveal a
Deficiency of Spleen Qi or Yang. If there are symptoms such as headaches, dizziness, anger or blurred
vision, then Heat in the Liver is diagnosed.

If the tongue is swollen with tooth marks along the
sides, this clearly shows a Deficiency of Spleen Qi.

THIN TONGUE

A thin tongue appears thinner than normal and even
slightly shrunken. Thinness indicates a lack of proper
Body Fluids; if the tongue is pale, Blood Deficiency is
the problem; a red, thin tongue discloses Yin
Deficiency. The tongue may also be dry.

SWELLING IN ONE AREA

Swelling in a particular part of the tongue indicates a
problem with the organ related to that region (see
diagram on *page 46*). Swollen edges, for example, suggests a Deficiency in the Spleen, while a swollen tip
can indicate a Heart problem. Swelling between the
tip and central area suggests a Lung problem.

INDENTATION IN ONE AREA

A depression or indentation in a particular area shows
a Deficiency in the related organ (see diagram on *page
46*). A tooth-marked tongue, sometimes called a scal-
loped tongue, can be due to Spleen Deficiency. If it is
abnormally stiff, it may suggest a Heart problem.

LONG TONGUE

A long, narrow tongue can indicate Heat and is also
often red in colour. This tongue shape is frequently
associated with Heat in the Heart and traditional
Chinese Medicine theory would suggest a constitu-
tional tendency towards Heart disease.

LEFT **By gauging the overall
shape of the tongue, and noting
features in specific areas, the
colour diagnosis can be refined.
A swollen tongue reveals Qi and
Yang are blocked, as if by a dam.**

TONGUE COATING

The coating of the tongue gives an accurate report on the state of all the organs, but particularly the organs of digestion. When observing the coating, we are looking at the colour, thickness, distribution and texture of the coat. However, the coating can be affected by consumption of certain foods, drinks or medicines, so should not be inspected shortly after taking any of these. The tongue coating may reflect the presence of a pathogen in the body, which will usually be seen as Phlegm or Dampness. A normal, healthy tongue should have a thin, white, and slightly moist coating. This is produced as a natural by-product of the digestive process.

COLOUR OF COATING

The colour of the coating reveals the nature of the problem (if any). A white coating indicates Cold, a yellow coating indicates Heat, and a dirty grey coating indicates Dampness or Food Stagnation.

THICKNESS OF COATING

The thickness of the coating lets us know how severe the problem is: the thicker the coat, the more Dampness or Phlegm is present.

DISTRIBUTION OF COATING

The distribution of the coating shows the location of the disharmony in the body.

ESSENTIALS

A tongue coating is normal. Any changes to the ideal thin white covering indicate disease.

The coating can be affected by food or smoking. The position of cracks and spots needs to be carefully noted.

ABSENCE OF COATING

An absence of coating, known as a stripped tongue, shows a lack of proper Body Fluids due to Yin Deficiency, and usually occurs on a red tongue. If there is no coating present on the entire tongue surface, it denotes a serious Yin Deficiency. More commonly, small patches of the tongue lack a coating, indicating a Yin Deficiency in the organ related to that area.

DRY/WET COATING

A dry coating means that either Heat, or a Deficiency of Qi or Yang, is present (differentiated by other symptoms). A wet coating, which may be greasy and sticky, proves a Dampness due to Cold.

RIGHT **A normal tongue retains a moist sheen, like oil on water.**

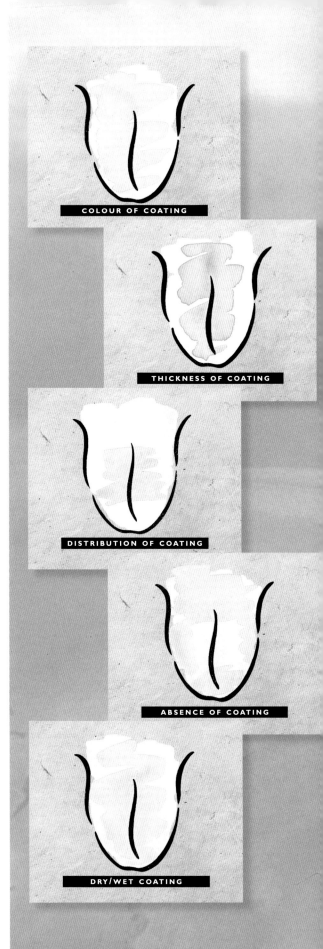

COLOUR OF COATING

THICKNESS OF COATING

DISTRIBUTION OF COATING

ABSENCE OF COATING

DRY/WET COATING

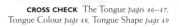

CRACKS

CRACKS AND SPOTS

Many types of alteration to the normal tongue surface are possible, and the significance of these is determined by their type and location.

CRACKS

The Chinese view of cracks on the tongue is related to the tongue as an expression of the moisture levels in the body. In the same way as the tongue swells if there is Excess Water (or Heat) present, a lack of Body Fluids may cause it to become cracked. Think of the way a dried-up river bed cracks after a drought.

Cracks are actual cuts in the tongue. (This should be distinguished from the rumpled appearance sometimes seen in a swollen tongue, resembling skin that has been in water for a long time.) Cracks can be found with or without a tongue coating, and their significances are combined if both are present.

LOCATION OF CRACKS

The significance of cracks is determined by their depth and location. The deeper the cracks, the more severe or long-standing the condition. The location indicates the problem organ.

🐟 Generalized small cracks over the tongue: Dryness of the Stomach and maybe Deficiency of Spleen Yin.

🐟 Severe cracking: Deficiency of Kidney Yin.

🐟 Vertical cracks on the sides of the tongue: Deficiency of the Spleen Qi or Yang. These will most often be found on a pale tongue.

🐟 A vertical crack down the centre of the tongue shows up a problem with the Stomach, or Heart and Stomach, depending on the length of the crack. A crack that does not extend to the tip (Heart area) indicates a Deficiency of the Stomach Yin. If the crack extends to the tip, and especially if there is a forking at the end of the tongue, there will be emotional problems related to the Heart.

SPOTS

Spots on the tongue can be found in different locations and in various colours. The location determines the organ involved; the colour reveals the problem.

Red spots indicate Heat, purple spots indicate Stagnation of Blood, and pale spots indicate Stagnation of Qi. The size and number of spots, as well as the depth of their colour, tells us the severity of the disharmony. Refer to the tongue diagram on page 46 to determine which organ is affected.

LEFT **Like a parched desert, the tongue can be covered with a network of cracks, indicating a lack of moisture.**

LOCATION OF CRACKS

SPOTS

The pulse

The other great pillar of Chinese diagnosis is the taking of the pulse. A full understanding of the significance of the pulse and its diagnostic potential takes a lifetime to master. However, it is possible to give a simplified overview of the things to look for when taking a pulse. When this simple version is used in conjunction with a tongue diagnosis, it will still allow you to ascertain much about the condition of your Qi and Blood.

The pulse can be taken at many sites on the body, but since Li Shi Zhen's ancient text *Classic of the Pulse*, physicians have standardized the taking of the pulse at the radial artery on the wrist.

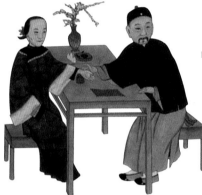

LEFT **An ancient Chinese painting depicting a court physician taking a woman's pulse.**

PHILOSOPHY

The concept of the pulse is quite different in Chinese Medicine. It is a way of coming directly into contact with the patient's Qi, as it is the Lungs that govern Qi through respiration. Great differences can be felt between the pulse in each wrist, which, interestingly, would be confirmed by a cardiologist.

THE NINE PULSES

An experienced practitioner of Chinese Medicine is able to locate nine different pulses on each wrist, giving a total of eighteen. The physician will use three fingers, carefully putting each on top of a different pulse. There are three levels to the pulse at each position, giving a total of nine pulses.

Each of the eighteen pulses is related to a specific internal organ, and gives detailed information about the state of that organ. Additionally, there are 28 pulse qualities that describe the state of the Qi. These translate into terms such as the Slippery Pulse, which indicates the presence of Dampness, or the Tight Pulse, which appears when there is obstruction. Any of the pulse qualities can be found at any of the pulse positions, and each signifies a different condition.

The eighteen pulses

RIGHT **In each of three positions on the wrist, there are three different levels of pulse, making a total of nine pulses. Adding both wrists together makes a total of eighteen pulses. Each area is linked to an organ. The Heart refers to organs and functions above the diaphragm (especially left side); the Liver to those between diaphragm and navel (especially lateral areas); the Kidney Yin to those below the navel (especially lower left).**

LEFT **The Lung correlates with organs and functions above the diaphragm (especially right side); the Spleen with those between diaphragm and navel (especially central); Kidney Yang with those below the navel (especially lower right).**

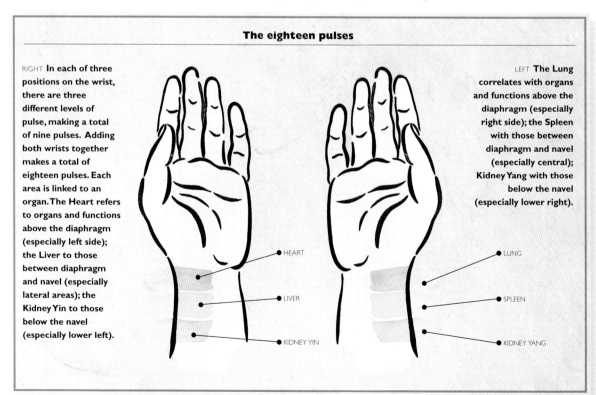

HEART

LIVER

KIDNEY YIN

LUNG

SPLEEN

KIDNEY YANG

How to feel the pulse

1 The person should be sitting opposite you, with hands held comfortably at around the level of the solar plexus or chest.

PLACE YOUR SECOND
FINGER JUST BELOW THE
WRIST CREASE

KEEP ARM
RELAXED

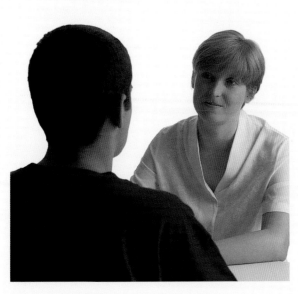

2 Use the fingers of your right hand to feel the person's left wrist, and vice versa.

PRESS GENTLY AND
EVENLY WITH ALL
THREE FINGERS

FEEL THE PULSE
FOR A MINUTE.
WHAT IS IT LIKE?

ESSENTIALS
The Zang-Fu organs are reflected in the eighteen pulses, which help pinpoint any imbalance.

The three different levels involved in pulse-taking reflect the different stages of a disease and the degree of imbalance.

3 Use the middle three fingers of your left hand to feel the right pulse. Place your second finger just below the person's wrist crease (on the thumb side) over the radial artery. Then allow the other two fingers to rest gently next to this. You should not use your thumb, as you may confuse your own pulse with that of the patient.

Press with all three fingers, evenly and gently, until you can just feel a pulse. Stay here for a minute and become aware of the quality of the pulse.

4 Press a little harder until the pulse disappears, then ease off very slightly until you can feel it again. Stay here for a minute, and see if you think the nature of the pulse at this deeper level is different in any way from the first pulse.

You have now felt the quality of the person's Qi.

WHAT TO LOOK FOR

Depth, Speed, and Strength are the aspects to look for. The healthy pulse is felt easily, and has a smooth and steady rhythm. It varies according to age, constitution and fitness. Generally, the pulse slows down with age and its strength will depend on build – a muscular man has a more forceful pulse than a thin woman. The pulse is not considered to be fully developed in children under seven, and a novice is unlikely to gain much useful information from a child's pulse.

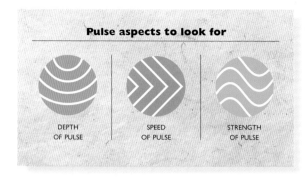

Pulse aspects to look for

DEPTH OF PULSE   SPEED OF PULSE   STRENGTH OF PULSE

Depth – a pulse can be Normal, Superficial, or Deep

● The Normal pulse should be easy to find, at all depths.

● The Superficial pulse is felt very easily with light pressure, but disappears on deep pressure. This pulse signifies that there is more Qi in the upper part of the body than the lower part. (This happens in Yin Deficiency of the Kidneys, causing headaches, tinnitus and hot flushes. It can also appear when there is too much energy in the Lungs, such as a cough or symptoms of asthma.)

● The Deep pulse is absent upon light palpation and is only felt on deep pressure. It indicates a Deficiency of Yang energy, as there is not enough Yang Qi to lift the pulse up to the surface. (Amongst other problems, this can lead to symptoms such as tiredness, prolapse, diarrhoea, incontinence and vaginal discharge.)

Speed – a pulse can be Normal, Rapid, or Slow

● The Normal pulse has a smooth, steady rhythm, neither fast nor slow.

● The Rapid pulse is faster than is normal for the patient's age. (This must be measured as the resting pulse. The pulse will be elevated if the person has just been active or is very anxious.)

The Rapid pulse indicates Heat, and the faster the pulse, the more Heat is present. The Heat can be of a Full or Empty nature, and this is differentiated by other signs and symptoms.

● The Slow pulse is slower than is normal for the patient's age. A Slow pulse indicates Cold, and the slower the pulse, the more Cold is present. This Cold can be of a Full or Empty nature, and this is ascertained from other signs and symptoms.

Strength – a pulse can be Normal, Full or Empty

● The pulse in the right wrist gives information mostly about the Qi, whereas the pulse in the left wrist is predominately Blood-oriented. If the Fullness or Emptiness is mostly on one side, then the organs which are affected are as follows:

Left: Liver, Heart, Kidney Yin.
Right: Spleen, Stomach, Lungs, Kidney Yang.

● The Full pulse is very forceful, with an aggressive wave quality. It will usually be felt easily on both levels, and with all three fingers. The more pronounced the force, the greater the degree of Fullness. A Full pulse reveals an Excess of something in the body, so the appropriate treatment is to determine and then clear it.

● The Empty pulse is weak, with a loose wave quality. The more pronounced the weakness, the more Empty the condition is. An Empty pulse marks a Deficiency of something in the body, so the appropriate treatment is to determine the area of weakness and then strengthen it.

Palpation

Various areas on the body are called Mu Xue, or alarm points. These warn of problems with organs. If there is tenderness when any of these regions are pressed, it tells us that the corresponding organ is disharmonious.

HOW TO PALPATE THE ORGAN ZONES

Using the fingers of one or both hands, press gently but firmly 2–7cm (1–3in) into the muscle. The number of fingers to use and the amount of pressure to apply will depend on the area palpated and the size of the patient. Fleshy areas on larger people will require more fingers and more pressure than small bony areas on thin people or children.

If marked tenderness is found at any of the Mu Xue, then you may have located a problem. You can now go on to ask other questions related to that organ in order to come to a diagnosis.

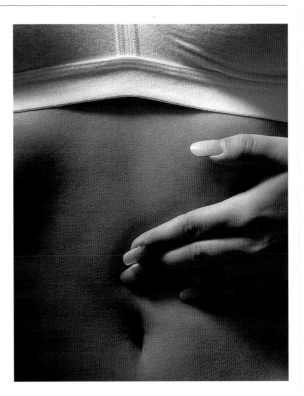

RIGHT **Palpating the zone relating to the Stomach, to look for tender areas on a patient who has complained of digestive problems.**

All sorts of touching

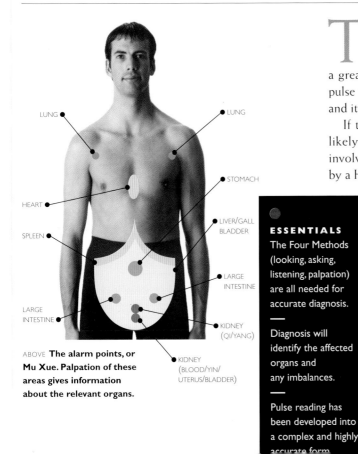

LUNG

LUNG

STOMACH

HEART

LIVER/GALL BLADDER

SPLEEN

LARGE INTESTINE

LARGE INTESTINE

KIDNEY (QI/YANG)

KIDNEY (BLOOD/YIN/ UTERUS/BLADDER)

ABOVE **The alarm points, or Mu Xue. Palpation of these areas gives information about the relevant organs.**

The fourth Chinese diagnostic tool, covering palpation and pulse-taking, is sometimes described as 'touching'. A physician can learn a great deal, not only from areas of tenderness and pulse patterns, but also from the body's temperature and its degree of dryness or level of moisture.

If the skin feels cold to the touch, then it is very likely that a Cold syndrome or Yang Deficiency is involved. If it feels hot, the problem may be caused by a Heat imbalance or a Yin Deficiency.

An excessively dry skin might be caused by a lack of Blood or Body Fluids, or possibly by Heat invading the Blood, as with some types of dry eczema. If the skin feels oily, this can suggest Dampness.

These indications, combined with the information gleaned from looking, asking and listening, give the physician an overall picture of the patient's health, and help to identify the disease syndrome involved.

We have looked at the ways of assessing the body's energy and health. To see how to put it all together, turn to *page 58.*

ESSENTIALS
The Four Methods (looking, asking, listening, palpation) are all needed for accurate diagnosis.

Diagnosis will identify the affected organs and any imbalances.

Pulse reading has been developed into a complex and highly accurate form

SELF-DIAGNOSIS

There are two main reasons for wanting to assess your health: either you have an existing disharmony that you want to treat, or you want to maintain your health at its present level. Either way, before any form of advice can be taken or any treatment followed, you must know where and what the actual or potential problem is. This simple questionnaire may help.

How to use this questionnaire

The questionnaire is a means of collating all the important information you will need to answer the questions you will ask yourself when reading through this book. You may well find that you need to add new information or refine your answers as you work through the text. Make several photocopies of the questionnaire to fill in.

Health assessment questionnaire

1 WHAT WOULD YOU SAY IS YOUR MAIN HEALTH PROBLEM?

2 DO YOU HAVE A DIAGNOSIS FROM YOUR DOCTOR?

3 IF THERE IS MORE THAN ONE PROBLEM, REPEAT THE QUESTIONS FOR EACH

- When did the problem first start?
- Where do the symptoms occur?
- Describe the main symptoms.
- Does anything make the symptoms worse?
- Does anything make the symptoms better?
- What treatment, if any, have you had for this problem?
- Does this problem relate to another health issue?
- In what way are they affected by each other?

ESSENTIALS
Diagnosis involves many probing questions to identify relevant symptoms.

Thirst levels, food preferences, or sleeping patterns can all help to identify a disharmony.

4 WATERWORKS

- Describe your usual thirst level.
- How much fluid do you drink in a day?
- Do you generally prefer hot drinks or cold drinks?
- How many times do you usually pass water in a day?
- How many times do you usually pass water at night?
- What are the colour and volume?
- Do you get any discomfort, difficulty or burning with urination?

5 ENERGY

- Describe how you feel most of the time.
- When are you most aware of feeling tired?
- How do you feel when you wake in the morning?

6 DIGESTION

- Describe your appetite.
- Do you get acidity? What causes it?
- Do you get bloating? What causes it?
- Do you get nausea? What causes it?
- Do you have any food intolerance? Specify which.
- Do you get food cravings? Specify which.

7 BOWEL MOVEMENTS

- *Are your bowel movements:*

  Daily? (How many times?)

  If not, how often? (Every ___ days.)

  Formed? Describe.

  Loose? Describe.

  Hard?

  Alternating between constipation and diarrhoea?

- *Is there any:*

  Pain?

  Blood?

  Mucus?

  Wind?

  Straining?

8 EATING HABITS

- How many times a day do you have a full meal?
- Do you snack?
- Do you regularly skip meals?
- Have you regularly been on a weight loss diet? (Specify which.)
- Do you tend to gain or lose weight more easily?
- Do you often eat at different times every day, or very late at night?
- Describe a typical breakfast.
- Describe a typical lunch.
- Describe a typical supper.
- What snacks or treats do you eat?
- Do you often need to rush, work or do something else during one of these meals?
- Note any foods that you know will probably bring on a particular symptom and describe the symptom.

9 PAIN

- Do you regularly get pain anywhere? (Specify where.)
- Describe the pain.
- Does it travel to any other location?
- What brings the pain on?
- What eases it?

10 FEMALE GYNAECOLOGY

- How old were you when you had your first period?
- What was it like when it started?
- What is the average time between periods now?
- If they are irregular, give the shortest and longest cycles.
- How long do your periods last?
- Which is the heaviest day(s)?
- Is there any pain? How severe is it?
- Describe the flow and how it changes (fresh, dark, clots, spotting, thin).
- Does your mood change before your period?
- Describe the mood changes. How long before your period do they start?
- Do you get any physical symptoms before your period begins?
- Have you ever been pregnant? If so, do you have any children?
- What were your pregnancies and labour like?
- What forms of contraception have you used?
- If you have been through the menopause, describe what it was like for you.

11 MENTAL / EMOTIONAL

- What word or phrase would you use to describe your mental and emotional states?
- Have you ever suffered from anxiety or depression?
- Do you regularly experience a particular type of uncontrollable emotion?
- What are your concentration and memory like?
- Do you have any problems getting to sleep?
- Do you wake at night?
- Do you have dreams that disturb your sleep?

12 GENERAL QUESTIONS

- Do you feel more sensitive to certain temperatures or weather? Specify.
- Do you get hot or sweat abnormally?
- Do you have any particular problems with your ears, eyes or nose? Describe.
- Describe any previous history of illness.
- Are there any hereditary diseases which run in your family? Specify which.
- Note down any medication or supplements that you take on a regular basis.

PUTTING IT ALL TOGETHER

A Chinese saying states: 'The skilful doctor treats those who are well, but the inferior doctor can only treat those who are ill.' Preventative medicine – understanding your own weaknesses and imbalances – has been central to Chinese theory for over 2,000 years.

How to conduct your self-diagnosis

Self-diagnosis is never simple and for serious or chronic conditions it is always best to consult a professional practitioner. For simple, self-limiting problems, following the sequence on the checklist on *pages 56–57* will help to indicate the cause of the imbalance. This is, of course, just a beginning. Chinese Medicine includes far more disease syndromes than those confined to Phlegm, Damp and Food Stagnation – although these are among the most common encountered in cool, damp, temperate climates. The Six Evils of Wind, Cold, Summer Heat, Dampness, Dryness and Fire (external causes of disease) can attack in combination, such as Damp-Cold or Phlegm-Heat. Wind-Damp, for example, is blamed for certain skin disorders. Fire often spreads to the internal organs; this is blamed for a range of illnesses that Western medicine may label as bronchitis or chronic gastritis. According to Chinese Medicine, arthritis is a combined attack by Wind, Cold and Damp. Sufferers often find that their symptoms are worse in cold, damp weather while sometimes – like the wind – the aches and twinges can move around the body affecting various joints at different times. These external factors can cause us all health problems from time to time and, if kept in check, these are often no more than minor, superficial complaints. Chinese Medicine believes in combating ills as early as possible, rather than waiting for conditions to deteriorate, when they will start to affect the balance of Qi and Yin-Yang.

Other ailments are caused by internal problems, such as a depletion of certain sorts of Qi as part of the natural ageing process; or by an imbalance in the Five Elements, leading to over-activity in some of the Zang-Fu organs and suppression of the functions of others. This is where it is useful to have previously identified your body type, so you are aware of the potential problems which might afflict you. By understanding your own internal balance, you can quickly spot changes and take some remedial action to prevent further deterioration.

BELOW **Working out a diagnosis is like putting building blocks together.**

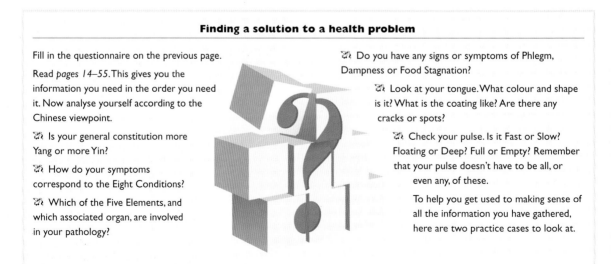

Finding a solution to a health problem

Fill in the questionnaire on the previous page.

Read *pages 14–55*. This gives you the information you need in the order you need it. Now analyse yourself according to the Chinese viewpoint.

🔖 Is your general constitution more Yang or more Yin?

🔖 How do your symptoms correspond to the Eight Conditions?

🔖 Which of the Five Elements, and which associated organ, are involved in your pathology?

🔖 Do you have any signs or symptoms of Phlegm, Dampness or Food Stagnation?

🔖 Look at your tongue. What colour and shape is it? What is the coating like? Are there any cracks or spots?

🔖 Check your pulse. Is it Fast or Slow? Floating or Deep? Full or Empty? Remember that your pulse doesn't have to be all, or even any, of these.

To help you get used to making sense of all the information you have gathered, here are two practice cases to look at.

OBSERVATIONS

Alicia's pulse was weak on the right, Full on the left. Tongue slightly pale, swollen, distinct tooth marks on the side. Sticky coating in the centre, few pale spots down both sides.

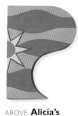

Applying the Eight Conditions

Are Alicia's symptoms due to Heat or Cold – is there too much of one and not enough of the other?

The symptoms are not simply Hot or Cold or predominately Yin or Yang in nature.

ABOVE **Alicia's symptoms do not reveal Heat or Cold.**

There is tiredness and she feels worse after diarrhoea, which suggests Emptiness. Constipation and PMS improve when her period starts, which suggests Fullness. The problem is chronic in nature and involves the organs, so it is an Interior condition.

Applying the Five Elements

Is a particular Element indicated in Alicia's case?

Earth governs the digestion via the Spleen and Stomach. Loose stools and diarrhoea are most commonly due to a Deficiency of Spleen Qi. This idea is reinforced by the symptoms of tiredness, poor memory and broken concentration.

Wood has an important effect on the periods and particularly on PMS. The Liver is associated with Wood and controls the movement of Qi

ABOVE **Alicia found that continual tiredness was making it difficult for her to work efficiently.**

LEFT **Lack of Spleen Qi is associated with the Earth Element.**

> **Alicia's case**
>
> **Patient:** Alicia, age 35. Works as a PA.
>
> **History:** Digestive problems for six years. Irritable bowel syndrome.
>
> **Symptoms:** Loose bowel movements two or three times daily, often mucus with the stools; occasional bouts of diarrhoea when very stressed, causing her to feel drained and tired. Constipation the week before her period – doesn't empty her bowels for up to four days, and then it is dry and painful. Bloating and severe, cramping abdominal pain which passes after a bowel movement or when period starts. Marked PMS symptoms such as mood swings and irritability. Over the last few years, periods have become more irregular. Tired a lot of the time, forgets things, lowered concentration. Often skips lunch or grabs a sandwich while working on the computer. Got out of the habit of breakfast years ago.

in the body, and therefore of Blood too. Irregular periods, changes in emotional state and lack of movement (constipation leading to abdominal pain), are all indicative of an inability on the part of the Liver to move the Qi and Blood smoothly.

Alicia's irregular eating habits over a period of several years have weakened her Spleen Qi. Refer to the section on Earth as the transitional season (*page 25*) to see the effects this can have on the digestion.

Looking for Phlegm, Dampness or Food Stagnation

Is there any evidence of Phlegm, Dampness or Food Stagnation?

Mucus in the stools usually indicates Phlegm and Dampness. The Spleen is the source of Phlegm and Dampness in the body. In Alicia's case, the Deficient Spleen Qi is allowing Dampness to form.

> **ESSENTIALS**
> Applying the diagnostic routine helps to pinpoint the problem.
>
> Lifestyle cannot be ignored. Energy imbalances can become manifest in unexpected ways.

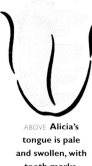

ABOVE **Alicia's tongue is pale and swollen, with tooth marks.**

☜ Reading the tongue

What does the tongue tell us?

The paleness and swelling indicate Deficiency of the Qi. The tooth marks on the side are particular to the Spleen. The sticky coating confirms the presence of Dampness and, as it is in the centre, this shows that it is located in the Spleen and Stomach. The spots down both sides of the tongue are over the Liver area, indicating a Stagnation of the Liver energy.

☜ Reading the pulse

What does the pulse signify?

The weak pulse on Alicia's right wrist tells us the Qi of the digestion, Spleen and Stomach is Deficient. The Full pulse on her left wrist shows that the state of the Blood and the Liver is tense.

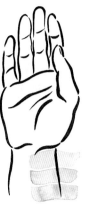

ABOVE **Alicia's right pulse shows a lack of Qi.**

Summary

Looking at Alicia's busy and stressful lifestyle, it is clear that her job and the demands it exerts on her has taken its toll. Alicia's poor eating habits over a period of years have damaged her digestive Qi. (This energy is the basis of healthy Blood. The Spleen and Stomach are responsible for turning food into Blood.)

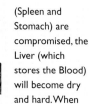

In Chinese Medicine, women's health is said to be dominated by Blood (and men's health by Qi). This refers to the importance of the Blood in roles such as fertility, pregnancy, periods and the menopause. If the sources of Blood production (Spleen and Stomach) are compromised, the Liver (which stores the Blood) will become dry and hard. When this happens, the Liver is unable to control the movement of Qi, and various symptoms of Fullness can arise. In Alicia's case these are constipation before her period, PMS, a Full pulse on the left wrist, spots down the sides of the tongue, and abdominal pain.

Deficient Spleen energy is evident from the diarrhoea, the tiredness, the inability to concentrate and her poor memory, her weight gain, a weak pulse on the right wrist, and a pale and tooth-marked tongue.

Patient: Suzie, aged 47, housewife, with two children aged 17 and 20.

History: Experiencing menopausal problems.

Symptoms: Suzie's periods started to become more irregular a couple of years ago. The gaps between them became longer and she would miss some altogether. This didn't particularly concern her and she just assumed it was her age until she started to get hot flushes. These would come on suddenly during the day, when she would become very hot and flushed, and break out into a sweat. As if this wasn't awkward enough, she started to become anxious in situations that would never have bothered her before and her sleep became more and more restless. She also found that sex was difficult because of vaginal dryness. Her doctor recommended that she start to take hormone replacement therapy (HRT), but she was reluctant to do this as she was concerned about the side-effects.

RIGHT **Although normally confident and optimistic, Suzie was finding her menopausal symptoms were undermining her feelings of well-being.**

OBSERVATIONS

Pulse slightly Rapid, Tense, felt easily with little pressure. Tongue red, dry, absence of normal coating.

🗱 Applying the Eight Conditions

Are Suzie's symptoms due to Heat or Cold – is there too much of one and not enough of the other?

After a lifetime of periods and having had children, it is natural that the Blood will become Deficient. As Blood is a Yin substance, this will often develop into Yin Deficiency over time. The relative lack of Yin in the

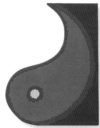

ABOVE **Yang is out of control, so Yin has become Deficient.**

body allows the heating nature of the Yang energy to become uncontrolled, which produces internal Heat and Dryness. This manifests in the dry eyes and dry vagina which occur in some menopausal women.

🗱 Applying the Five Elements

Is a particular Element indicated in Suzie's case?

The two main expressions of Yin and Yang energy in the body are the polar forces of Fire and Water. These two should be in harmony, so the Water does not quench the Fire, and the Fire does not damage the Water. With Suzie, the Water Element is weak, which allows the Fire to become uncontrolled. In terms of the organs, this relates to the Water organ of the Kidney and the Fire organ of the Heart. If there is too much Heat in the Heart, the Shen-Mind becomes restless and anxiety and poor sleep will result. Inherited Qi, stored in the Kidneys, gradually runs down during the course of a person's life.

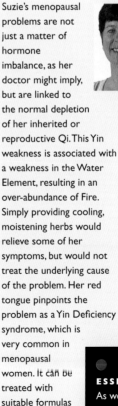

ABOVE **Suzie's inherited Qi is low, and Water is weak.**

Women's lives are traditionally measured in seven-year spans and by the age of 49 this Kidney Qi is nearly exhausted, adding to the general weakness of the organ.

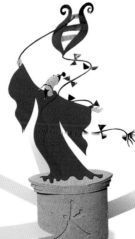

RIGHT **Suzie has too much Heat, causing problems in the Heart, which is associated with the Fire Element.**

🗱 Looking for Phlegm, Dampness or Food Stagnation

Is there any evidence of Phlegm, Dampness or Food Stagnation? None of these noted.

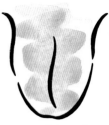

ABOVE **A dry, red tongue: Heat and a lack of Yin.**

🗱 Reading the tongue

What does the tongue tell us? A red tongue tells us that Heat is present. It is dry with no coating, indicating a lack of Yin.

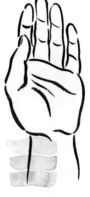

🗱 Reading the pulse

What does the pulse signify? This type is called a Floating pulse, because it can be felt straight away, but disappears on pressure. This is because the Excess of Yang energy takes the Qi to the surface, as there is insufficient Yin to root the energy.

LEFT **A Floating pulse reveals dissipation of Qi.**

Summary

Suzie's menopausal problems are not just a matter of hormone imbalance, as her doctor might imply, but are linked to the normal depletion of her inherited or reproductive Qi. This Yin weakness is associated with a weakness in the Water Element, resulting in an over-abundance of Fire. Simply providing cooling, moistening herbs would relieve some of her symptoms, but would not treat the underlying cause of the problem. Her red tongue pinpoints the problem as a Yin Deficiency syndrome, which is very common in menopausal women. It can be treated with suitable formulas and tonic herbs such as He Shou Wu and Shu Di Huang. Using cooling herbs (to combat the flaring of Fire) with herbs to nourish the Blood and Yin replenishes the Kidney energy and controls the over-exuberance of Yang. Fire is, of course, related to the Heart, so excessive activity here can lead to Heart energy disturbances such as the emotional upsets, irritability and restlessness which some women may experience during the menopause.

ESSENTIALS
As well as external factors, internal problems need to be considered. To reach an accurate diagnosis, inherited and parental Qi aspects must be taken into account.

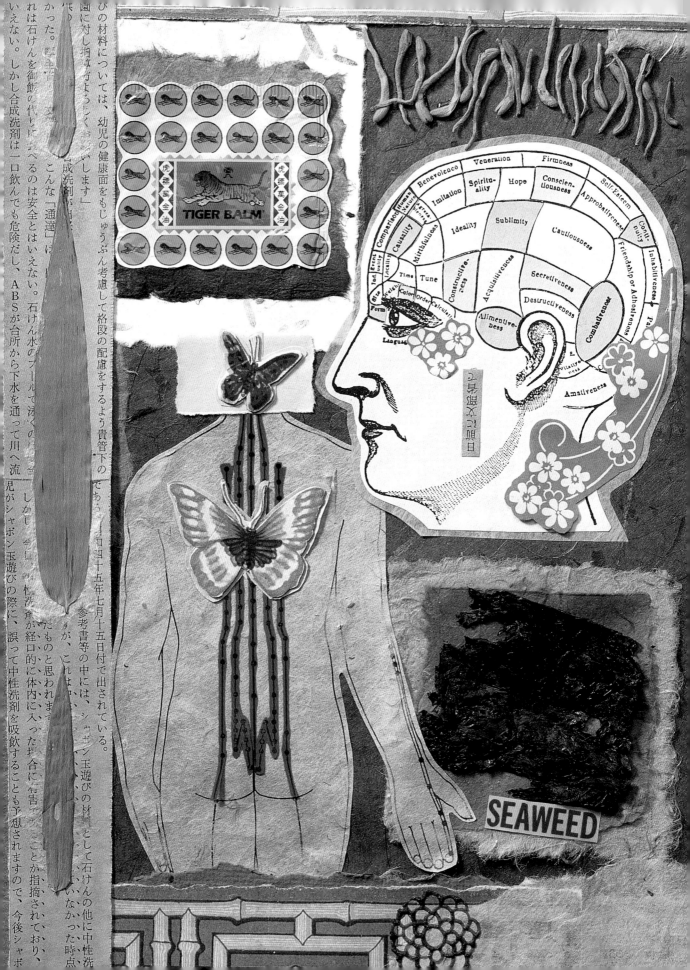

PART TWO

HOW HERBS
CAN HELP

In this section we will start to look at how you can use the information you have gathered about yourself to begin actual self-treatment. By following the diagnostic and assessment procedures in Part One, you should be able to establish which body system or organ is in disharmony. The next step is to refer to the relevant part in this section, working out which of the syndromes fit your particular pattern of symptoms.

MOXA ROLLS

TIGER BALM

TIGER BALM

TIGER BALM

HOW TO TREAT THE INDIVIDUAL ORGANS

As we saw in Part One, the internal organs are viewed quite differently in Chinese Medicine. The twelve organs are divided into pairs of Yin and Yang organs, two for each of the Five Elements, making ten. These are classed as solid (Zang) or hollow (Fu), and are collectively called Zang-Fu. The two additional 'organs' are really metaphors for body functions: the Triple Heater (San Jiao), which controls the distribution of Heat and Water around the body, and the Pericardium (Xin Bao), the outer protective layer of the Heart.

Organ functions

Yang organs are functional hollow workhouses (such as the Stomach, Intestines or Bladder), where crude Body Fluids are processed. The Yin organs (such as the Liver, Heart and Lungs), are solid organs where more precious fluids are stored.

When thinking about treating yourself with Chinese Medicine, it is important to remember that the Chinese view of anatomy is partially poetic. The organs are viewed on a functional rather than a literal basis, a system crafted from careful observation of the body, in health and disease, over thousands of years.

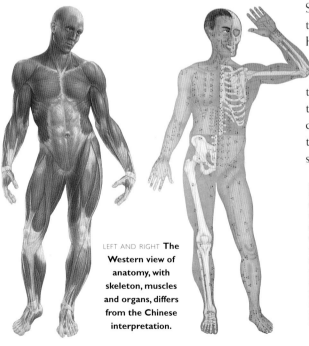

LEFT AND RIGHT **The Western view of anatomy, with skeleton, muscles and organs, differs from the Chinese interpretation.**

WHICH ORGANS ARE IMPORTANT?

You will find that some organs, which are seen as relatively unimportant in conventional Western medicine, have a critical role in Chinese Medicine. Likewise, organs that are frequently diagnosed as dysfunctional in conventional Western medicine are hardly discussed at all in traditional Chinese texts.

For instance, Western medicine regards the spleen as a largely superfluous organ, which can be removed without complications (although this view is now changing). In Chinese Medicine, however, the Spleen occupies a central role in all the transformative functions of the body, and is essential to health. However, little mention is made of the appendix, thyroid or pancreas in Chinese texts, although they are clearly important organs. This is because the functions of these glands and organs are under the jurisdiction of one of the twelve organs. The pancreas is considered part of the Spleen system, the thyroid part of the Kidney network, and so on. Each system works consistently within its own boundaries.

How to use this section

Use the information you have already gathered about yourself and check it against the symptoms for the body system you are trying to treat. This will tell you which organ pattern is involved, and you can then look it up in the formulas listed in Part Four.

MIND AND BODY

The Chinese have never regarded the mind and body as separate entities. This agrees with what we all already know: emotional stress can cause or worsen physical symptoms, and illness can affect us emotionally. In Chinese Medicine, when a body system, organ or Element is treated, the treatment is effective on all levels, not just the physical – the remedy has emotional and spiritual dimensions. You will see this holistic idea running throughout the treatment sections in this book, and it will help you to understand how your overall health is affected.

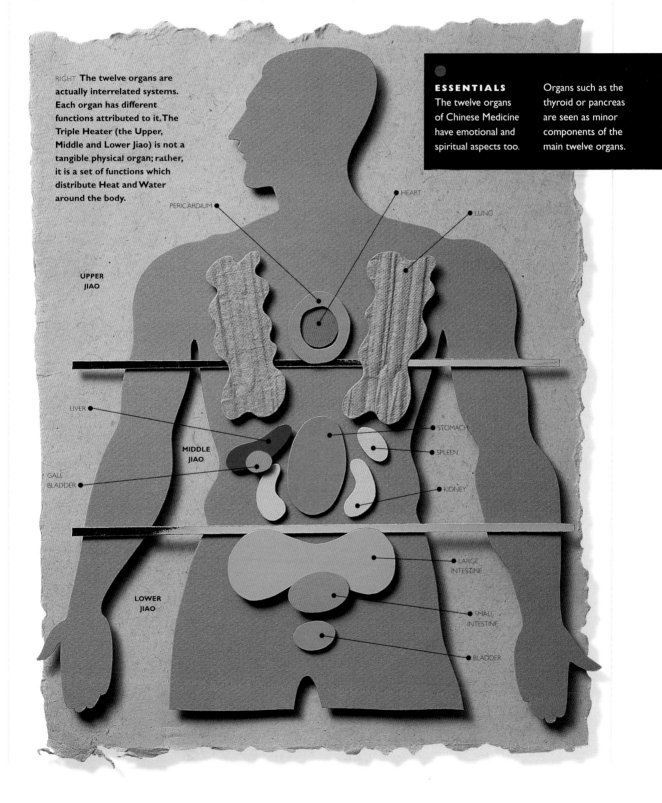

RIGHT **The twelve organs are actually interrelated systems. Each organ has different functions attributed to it. The Triple Heater (the Upper, Middle and Lower Jiao) is not a tangible physical organ; rather, it is a set of functions which distribute Heat and Water around the body.**

ESSENTIALS
The twelve organs of Chinese Medicine have emotional and spiritual aspects too.

Organs such as the thyroid or pancreas are seen as minor components of the main twelve organs.

PERICARDIUM

HEART

LUNG

UPPER JIAO

LIVER

STOMACH

MIDDLE JIAO

SPLEEN

GALL BLADDER

KIDNEY

LOWER JIAO

LARGE INTESTINE

SMALL INTESTINE

BLADDER

DIGESTIVE SYSTEM

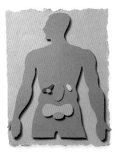

ABOVE **The Liver, Gall Bladder, Stomach, Spleen and Intestines make up the digestive system.**

An efficient digestive system is absolutely central to good health. It transforms the food you eat and the fluids you drink into Qi energy and Blood nourishment. With a good digestion, you will have lots of energy, and keep your body in good working order. If you do get ill, you will be more likely to recover from illness quickly. If the system is not fully functional, then imbalances in the distribution of the beneficial Jing, or 'essence' — distilled from food — can lead to problems.

The food route

The gastrointestinal tract is one continuous system from the mouth to the rectum. Food and fluids enter and are chopped up by the teeth and sent down to the Stomach, which is likened to a cooking pot with some water in it. The Spleen provides the fuel under the pot; the Liver and Gall Bladder add 'spices', in the form of bile. In the cooking pot, foods and liquids are turned into a soup.

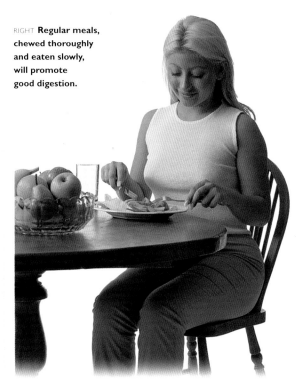

RIGHT **Regular meals, chewed thoroughly and eaten slowly, will promote good digestion.**

The soup is distilled into the Pure and the Impure. The Pure rises upwards to the Heart and Lungs, where it is circulated around the body by respiration. The Impure is drained out into the Intestines where some further extraction of nutrients takes place. The remaining matter is excreted by the Large Intestine as faeces. The main food nutrients are transformed into Blood, which is stored in the Heart and Liver.

THE FORMATION OF DAMPNESS AND PHLEGM

Damp and Phlegm can be produced at any stage of the digestive process if there is a breakdown in the system. If the food is not chopped up properly (insufficient chewing), the food will be too big for the pot. If there is not enough or too much water (Stomach Dryness or Dampness) in the pot, then the food will either be too wet or will burn. If the cooking heat is too low (Spleen Deficiency), the food will not cook properly. If no (or too many) 'spices' are used (Liver Stagnation, Gall Bladder Damp-Heat) then the meal will either be hard to digest or will cause indigestion. If the ingredients are not balanced, the meal will lack an appetizing aroma and nourishment. Qi will not be available to the Lungs, or Blood to the Heart.

Sticky deposits will build up if your body is not functioning well. In the middle and lower parts of the body such as the Spleen, Stomach, Bladder and Intestines these are referred to as Dampness. In the upper body, such as the Lungs, the deposits are called Phlegm (*see pages 42–45*).

Digestive system problems

SPLEEN AND STOMACH DEFICIENCY

Symptoms: Low energy, loose bowels or diarrhoea, poor concentration and thinking, irregular appetite and sweet cravings, heavy sensations in the muscles and body, bloating and tiredness after eating, nausea, weight gain, fluid retention, mild indigestion.

Tongue: Pale, swollen, wet coat.

Pulse: Empty.

Herbs: Strengthen Earth decoction.

STOMACH HEAT

Symptoms: Ravenous appetite but failure to put on weight, burning indigestion, hyperactivity, constipation, high thirst, craving for spicy food and stimulants (which may worsen symptoms).

Tongue: Red, dry, cracks in centre, yellow coat in centre.

Pulse: Rapid, Full.

Herbs: Nourish the Stomach decoction.

SPLEEN DAMPNESS

Symptoms: Muzzy head and dull headaches, cloudy thought processes, weight gain, aching muscles and limbs, nasal congestion, frequent nausea (may vomit phlegm), diarrhoea with mucus, poor appetite, lethargy and weakness, abdominal fullness, occasional dizziness.

Tongue: Pale, swollen, tooth-marked, greasy coating.

Pulse: Empty or Full.

Herbs: Clear the Spleen decoction.

LIVER AND SPLEEN DISHARMONY

Symptoms: Alternating constipation and diarrhoea, attacks of abdominal pain and vomiting when under stress, bloating and distension of the stomach, abdomen and flanks, emotional changes, indigestion and fluctuations in appetite.

Tongue: Pale if Spleen Deficiency predominates, red or purple if Liver Stagnation predominates.

Pulse: Full during an attack, Empty at other times.

Herbs: Harmonize Wood and Earth decoction.

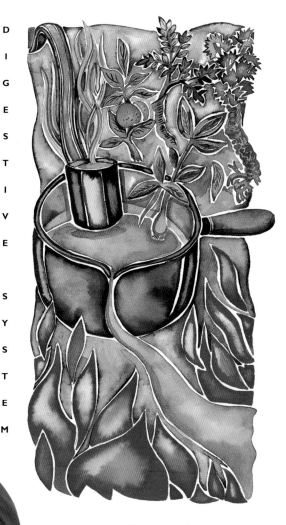

ABOVE **The process of digestion is like the cooking of a meal; the Stomach is represented by a cooking pot in which foods and liquids are turned into soup, which is then distilled into the Pure and Impure.**

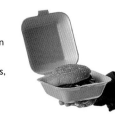

LEFT **Fast foods are often lacking in nutritional value, and may cause Damp, bringing on bloating and indigestion.**

ESSENTIALS

Eat regular, balanced meals for a healthy digestive system.

Poor diet soon upsets the energy levels of the main organs and can lead to Dampness and Phlegm.

Phlegm and Damp can interfere with the circulation of Qi.

WATER METABOLISM

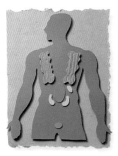

ABOVE **The Lungs, Stomach, Spleen, Kidneys and Bladder metabolize fluids.**

Your body is about 70 per cent water, just like the surface of the Earth. Fluids are essential to all bodily functions as they provide moisture, nourishment and cooling. In Chinese Medicine, Water metabolism in the body is governed by the three systems of the Triple Heater, or San Jiao. Each system – the Upper, Middle and Lower Jiao – deals with a different area of the body and ensures that food essences are properly separated and the fluids distributed to the correct tissues.

The fluid route

Fluids enter the Stomach where they are processed with the help of the Spleen. Water needs Heat to be transformed. The Yang energy of the Kidneys provides the Heat for all the transformative functions of the body. This Heat acts on the fluids and they are distilled into pure fluids that rise up to the Lungs (the Pure), and thick fluids that descend to the Kidneys and Bladder. Here, further separation takes place and the waste (the Impure) is excreted by the Bladder. The Lungs distribute the processed fluids to the skin, where some is lost as sweat, and send the rest to the Channels and organs.

TRIPLE HEATER SAN JIAO
The pathways through which these processes take place are described as the Triple Heater, or San Jiao. This is a way of dividing the body into the three areas where fluid transformations occur. The Upper Jiao (described as clouds) consists of the Lungs, Heart, head, chest, diaphragm and arms. The Middle Jiao (referred to as a bubbling cauldron) is the Stomach, Spleen, Liver, Gall Bladder, epigastrium and hypochondrium. The Lower Jiao (termed a drainage ditch) is the Kidneys, Bladder, Large Intestine, Small Intestine, uterus, legs and genitals.

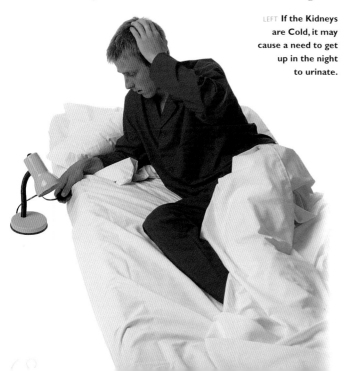

LEFT **If the Kidneys are Cold, it may cause a need to get up in the night to urinate.**

ESSENTIALS

Fluids are processed through a complex pathway which involves all three levels of the San Jiao.

Fluids in the Stomach are separated into Pure substances, sent to the Lungs, and Impure fluids, which are excreted.

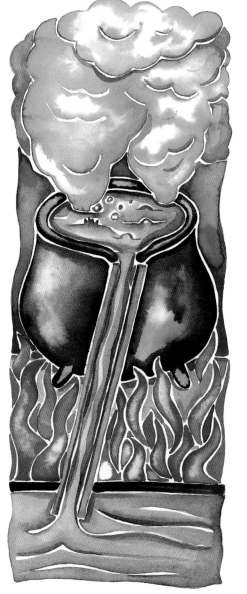

ABOVE **The Middle Jiao –
which includes the Stomach,
Spleen, Liver and Gall
Bladder – is like a bubbling
cauldron, from which Pure
fluids rise to the Upper Jiao,
and Impure fluids are
excreted through the
Lower Jiao.**

LEFT **The fluids
you drink pour
into the Stomach,
where they start
to be processed.**

M I D D L E   J I A O

Water metabolism problems

LOWER JIAO
KIDNEYS COLD

Symptoms: Frequent urination of lots of clear fluid, the
need to urinate at night, chronic low backache, feeling cold,
water retention in the lower body, pale complexion.

Tongue: Pale, swollen, white coat.

Pulse: Empty, Deep.

Herbs: Strengthen the Kidney decoction.

KIDNEYS HOT

Symptoms: Scanty dark urine, dull low backache, feeling
hot and sweaty, thirsty, flushed cheeks.

Tongue: Red, dry, may have peeled patches.

Pulse: Rapid, Empty, Superficial.

Herbs: Nourish the Kidney decoction.

DAMP-COLD IN THE BLADDER

Symptoms: Urinary urgency and frequency, feeling of
pressure and heaviness over bladder, difficulty in urinating,
urine pale and cloudy.

Tongue: White coat at back of tongue.

Pulse: Full.

Herbs: Drain the Bladder decoction.

DAMP-HEAT IN THE BLADDER

Symptoms: Urinary urgency and frequency, urination
interrupted or painful, dark and cloudy urine, possibly with
blood, fever (in severe cases).

Tongue: Yellow coat at back of tongue.

Pulse: Rapid, Full.

Herbs: Clear the Bladder decoction.

MIDDLE JIAO
SPLEEN DEFICIENCY

Symptoms: Bloating of the abdomen, swollen breasts,
nausea or poor appetite, diarrhoea, tiredness.

Tongue: Pale, swollen.

Pulse: Empty.

Herbs: Clear the Spleen decoction.

UPPER JIAO
LUNG DEFICIENCY

Symptoms: Shortness of breath, many colds, mucus,
stuffy or tight feeling in chest, cough, sneezing or wheezing,
feeling the cold, puffy face or hands, pale complexion.

Tongue: Pale.

Pulse: Empty.

Herbs: Strengthen Earth and Metal decoction.

HEART AND RESPIRATION

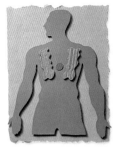

ABOVE **The Heart and Lungs are responsible for circulating Qi and Blood around the body.**

There are two main organs in the Upper Jiao: the Heart and Lungs. They work together to govern breathing and the circulation of Qi and Blood around the body. The Heart has a particular action on the Blood, and the Lungs on the Qi. They both have a separate and distinct rhythmic motion, which is responsible for the propulsion of the Qi and Blood around the body, and particularly throughout the network of Meridians or Channels.

Protection

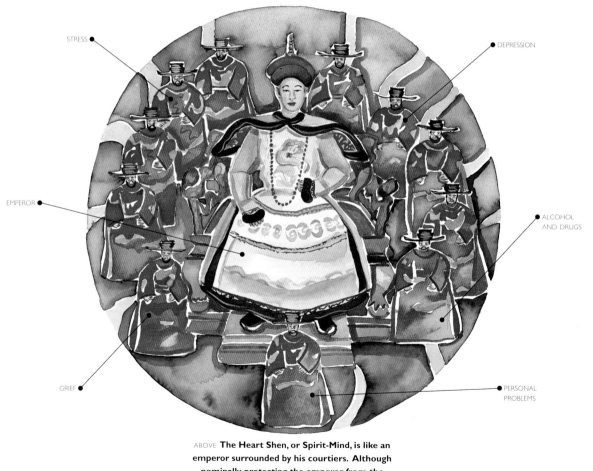

STRESS

DEPRESSION

EMPEROR

ALCOHOL AND DRUGS

GRIEF

PERSONAL PROBLEMS

ABOVE **The Heart Shen, or Spirit-Mind, is like an emperor surrounded by his courtiers. Although nominally protecting the emperor from the outside world, some courtiers may be plotting against him. These negative influences can weaken the Heart Shen.**

The Lungs correspond to many aspects of what we refer to in the West as the immune system. The Lungs are a Yin, Metal organ, thereby having protective qualities. They circulate the Wei Qi (Defensive Qi) to the outer muscle layer and open and close the skin pores, controlling the body's ability to protect itself from external invasion by pathogens. They also rule the nose – a weak Lung energy can be detected in those who react to airborne allergens such as pollen.

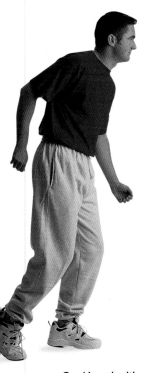

ABOVE **Good Lung health allows participation in aerobic sports such as jogging or tennis.**

THE SPIRIT

The Heart is described as an emperor, with the other eleven organs as his ministers. This supremacy confers on the Heart the role of housing the Shen (Spirit-Mind).

The Shen is said to be your consciousness – your personal soul, if you like. Your Shen makes you the individual person you are. However, just like an emperor, the Shen needs to be protected from the outside world, and is susceptible to negative influences. The Shen is easily injured by exposure to shock, emotional strain or an excess of stimulants. When this happens, the Shen loses its ability to remain calm, and insomnia, anxiety, erratic behaviour and nervousness may result. This will be covered in more detail in the section on emotional issues.

ESSENTIALS

The Heart and Lungs help circulate Qi and Blood.

—

The Heart governs the other organs.

—

Shen (Spirit-Mind) resides in the Heart; disturbance to it leads to anxiety and erratic behaviour.

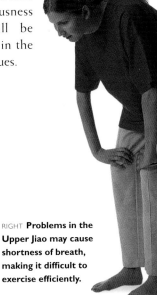

RIGHT **Problems in the Upper Jiao may cause shortness of breath, making it difficult to exercise efficiently.**

Upper Jiao problems

LUNG DEFICIENCY

Symptoms: Shortness of breath, catching colds easily, stuffy or tight feeling in chest, coughs, sneezing or wheezing, feeling the cold, pale complexion, spontaneous sweating, cold hands, tiredness.

Tongue: Pale.

Pulse: Empty.

Herbs: Strengthen Earth and Metal decoction.

LUNG PHLEGM-DAMPNESS

Symptoms: Cough with lots of white phlegm, nasal congestion, stuffy chest, shortness of breath.

Tongue: Thick white or grey coating.

Pulse: Full.

Herbs: Clear the Spleen or Dry the Lung decoction.

LUNG HEAT-DAMPNESS

Symptoms: Cough with lots of yellow-green sticky phlegm, coloured or bloody nasal discharge, stuffy chest, shortness of breath, wheezing.

Tongue: Thick, greasy, yellow coat.

Pulse: Rapid, Full.

Herbs: Clear the Lung decoction.

LUNG HEAT AND DRYNESS

Symptoms: Dry cough, shortness of breath, wheezing, sticky hard chest phlegm (may be blood-streaked), thirst, dry skin, red rash, flushed cheeks, dry-type constipation.

Tongue: Dry, red, thin, cracks in Lung area. May have thin, yellow coating.

Pulse: Rapid, Full.

Herbs: Moisten Metal decoction.

HEART DEFICIENCY

Symptoms: Palpitations, tiredness, shortness of breath on exertion, pale sallow complexion, insomnia, excess dreaming, anxiety.

Tongue: Pale, thin, may have a crack in the tip.

Pulse: Empty.

Herbs: Nourish the Heart decoction.

HEART HEAT

Symptoms: Palpitations, agitation, anxiety, insomnia, red complexion or red cheeks, dark urine, thirst, mouth or tongue ulcers.

Tongue: Red tip, possibly with central crack to tip.

Pulse: May be Full or Empty depending on severity, Rapid.

Herbs: Nourish and Calm the Heart decoction.

SKIN, HAIR AND NAILS

As external aspects of the body, the condition of the skin, hair and nails is dependent on nourishment from the Blood. They are all said to be made from the 'excess' of the Blood, so you can also guess at your Blood's richness from the state of these tissues. They are also linked to the Five Element model and can signify the underlying balance of their associated Zang organs. Skilled Chinese physicians can often make an accurate diagnosis simply by looking at these external tissues.

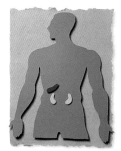

ABOVE **Kidneys and Liver affect skin, hair and nails.**

Maintenance

ESSENTIALS
The condition of skin, hair and nails reflects the state of the Kidneys and the Liver.

These organs are all closely linked to the Blood, so herbs to cool or nourish the Blood may be used.

BELOW **Using moisturizing creams and drinking plenty of water helps to rehydrate dry skin.**

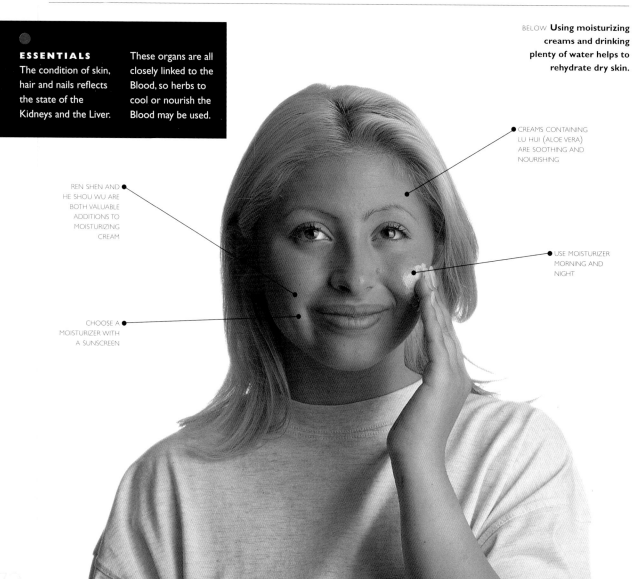

CREAMS CONTAINING LU HUI (ALOE VERA) ARE SOOTHING AND NOURISHING

REN SHEN AND HE SHOU WU ARE BOTH VALUABLE ADDITIONS TO MOISTURIZING CREAM

USE MOISTURIZER MORNING AND NIGHT

CHOOSE A MOISTURIZER WITH A SUNSCREEN

RIGHT **From soft, smooth and delicate, to wrinkles and 'character', the ageing of our skin is inevitable. But to a certain extent, we can improve its appearance by taking care of it.**

The skin relates to Metal (the skin is the third Lung) and to the Yin Blood. Deficiency or Dryness of either Metal energy or Blood can lead to a rough, cracked or wrinkled skin texture.

The hair is a direct reflection of Kidney energy, as it is considered an offshoot of the Kidney Essence, along with other tissues such as the bone marrow.

The nails are considered to be an extension of the tendons, and are therefore related to the Liver Blood.

Strengthening the Blood will have a beneficial effect on all of these tissues, and special attention can be paid to any organ that is particularly affected.

Problems with skin, hair and nails

GENERAL DRYNESS OF THE SKIN, HAIR AND NAILS

Symptoms: Dry, rough or cracked skin, dry and itchy skin rashes, flaky, ridged or cracked nails, dry or poor-quality hair.

Tongue: Pale, dry.

Pulse: Empty.

Herbs: Nourish the Blood decoction.

DRY AND IRRITATED SKIN

Symptoms: Skin that is more than just dry: there is a tendency to very dry, scaly or irritated itchy skin patches.

Tongue: May be red.

Pulse: Variable.

Herbs: Nourish and Cool the Blood decoction. (Not to be used for skin conditions where there are blisters or weeping fluid.)

SPOTS AND WET SKIN RASHES THAT WEEP FLUID

Symptoms: When toxins accumulate in the body, one of the ways in which they are cleared is via the skin, and this can be expressed as pus-filled spots or itchy patches that exude a clear or yellow fluid. Use the following herbal formula or follow the detoxification programme on *pages 94–95.* Toxin-clearing herbs are hard on the digestion, so you should not take this formula indiscriminately or for periods of more than one month at a time.

Tongue: May have a thick greasy coating.

Pulse: Variable.

Herbs: Clear Toxins from the Skin decoction.

DRY HAIR

Symptoms: Hair that is thin, brittle, dry and going prematurely grey.

Herbs: Nourish the Blood decoction.

DRY NAILS

Symptoms: Thin, cracked, ridged and brittle nails.

Herbs: Nourish the Blood decoction.

REHYDRATION

It is vital to keep up the Water content of the Blood if you suffer from Dryness. Consume plenty of water and herb tea, and avoid fluids that are dehydrating such as alcohol, tea and coffee.

EXTERNAL PREPARATIONS

There are a number of preparations which can be made to put on the skin or hair. Read about these in Part Four.

PAIN AND STIFFNESS

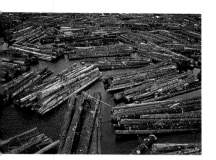

ABOVE **Pain often builds up gradually until it creates a log jam. Aches and twinges may lead to immobilizing pain if not tackled early.**

Pain is probably the single most common complaint that people suffer from, in every country in the world. Although there are many reasons for pain, in Chinese Medicine all pain is said to result from a blockage of Qi and Blood in the Meridian Channels, causing obstruction which results in Stagnation. Therefore, pain can always be treated by regulating and encouraging the flow of Qi and Blood.

Types of body pain

Chinese Medicine identifies various types of pain, which alert the physician to underlying problems. Distending pain is often due to Stagnating Qi, while a burning pain may be caused by Fire or Yang Heat from Yin Deficiency. Dull pain points to an imbalance in Qi and Blood flow. Asking questions about the quality of pain is an important part of Chinese diagnosis. The herbs suggested will depend on the area affected and the nature of the pain. The tongue and pulse will vary with these problems, according to the patient's general body type and constitution.

REFERRED PAIN FELT ALONG A CHANNEL

HEAVY, DULL, NAGGING ACHE JOINTS, BACK, NECK

THROBBING PAIN HEAD, FLANKS, ABDOMEN

STABBING PAIN JOINTS, MUSCLES, HEAD, LIMBS

INFLAMMATION ANY JOINT, COMMONLY THE FINGERS

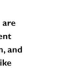

SWELLING JOINTS, INJURIES ANYWHERE

NUMBNESS / PINS AND NEEDLES LIMBS

GENERAL ACHING ANYWHERE

ESSENTIALS

An accurate description of the characteristics or type of pain helps to reveal its cause.

Pain is often associated with Qi or Blood Stagnation and can be eased by improving the flow of both.

RIGHT **There are many different types of pain, and they can strike at different sites on the body.**

Types of body pain

HEAVY AND STIFF

Symptoms: A dull, nagging ache. Will often be worse in humid or damp weather, and in the mornings. Improves after movement and with the application of heat or a hot shower. Can be severe and tight.

Indications: Cold-Dampness in the Channels.

Locations: Joints, back, neck.

Herbs: Warm the Channels decoction.

DULL

Symptoms: Generalized aching, which is neither sharp nor throbbing. Worse when tired or hungry, better after rest and after eating. Benefits from massage and pressure.

Indications: Pain from Deficiency of Qi or Blood.

Locations: Anywhere.

Herbs: Strengthen the Channels decoction.

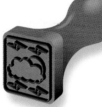

STABBING OR PIERCING

Symptoms: Localized severe pain. May be too sensitive to touch. Nothing seems to help.

Indications: Qi and Blood Stagnation.

Locations: Joints, muscles, head or limbs.

Herbs: Modified Regulate the Blood decoction (add Ji Xue Teng and Yan Hu Suo).

DISTENDING OR THROBBING

Symptoms: A bursting type of sensation where there is a feeling of pressure pushing from the inside outwards. The actual level of pain is dependent on the severity of the condition, and it may vary from mild to extreme.

Indications: Qi Stagnation.

Locations: Head, flanks, abdomen.

Herbs: For the head, use modified Free the Liver decoction (see Headaches); for the flanks or abdomen, use Harmonize Wood and Earth decoction.

NUMBNESS AND PINS AND NEEDLES

Symptoms: Both are caused by a lack of circulation to an area, but due to different reasons. Numbness results when there is Blood Deficiency causing lack of nourishment in an area, and it may be accompanied by cramps. Pins and needles occurs when there is a Channel obstruction stopping the Qi from getting to the extremities.

Locations: Limbs.

Herbs: For Blood Deficiency, use modified Nourish the Blood decoction (add Ji Xue Teng, increase dosage of Bai Shao by half). For Channel obstruction, use Strengthen the Channels decoction.

INFLAMMATION

Symptoms: Localized inflammation of the joints with redness and pain. Often accompanied by systemic symptoms such as changes in blood count or fever. Will usually be worse if alcohol or stimulants are consumed.

Indications: Heat, Yin Deficiency.

Locations: Any joint, but most commonly fingers.

Herbs: Modified Nourish the Kidney decoction (add Dan Shen).

REFERRAL OF PAIN

Symptoms: Pain can be felt along a Channel either at the area of blockage, or some distance from the site of the problem. Either way, the Channel that requires treatment can be isolated by matching the pain pathway with one of the Channels on the diagram on *page 17*.

Locations: Any of the twelve Channels, but most commonly the Yang Channels.

Herbs: Strengthen the Channels decoction, Warm the Channels decoction.

SWELLING

Swelling is a sign of local Stagnation, and can be due to Heat or Cold. If the skin is puffy, and neither red nor hot to the touch, the swelling is due to Cold and Damp. If there is marked inflammation with redness and a sensation of local heat, then Heat is the cause. It is important to differentiate between these two as hot packs should only be applied to Cold injuries; the reverse is of course true for Heat injuries.

Headaches

Billions of pounds are spent every year on drugs to cure headaches, but in fact you can treat many of them naturally by yourself. As well as herbs, diet plays an important role in the prevention of headaches, and certain foods may have to be eliminated if you want to get rid of the pain for good. When working out what type of headache you get, you will need to consider two main aspects – its location and the type of pain experienced.

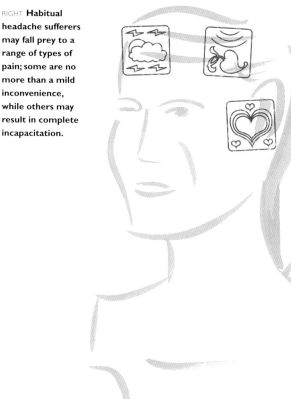

RIGHT **Habitual headache sufferers may fall prey to a range of types of pain; some are no more than a mild inconvenience, while others may result in complete incapacitation.**

MASSAGE

Massage of acupoints around the head, face and neck can be an excellent way of alleviating a headache. You don't need to know where the acupoints are, although you can get a chart from a Chinese Medical supplier if you are interested. Basically, if it hurts, rub it! If you get a regular headache, you will know where the pain is likely to travel to. Locate these areas with your fingertips and press firmly until you get a dull aching sensation. Hold or massage in small circles until the pain eases. Repeat this procedure for all painful areas.

You can also use a balm such as Tiger Balm to rub into the temples, forehead or neck. Be careful, however, as most balms contain ingredients such as menthol, which can irritate sensitive skin. Tiger Balm does not contain any tiger parts.

CAUTION

Headaches can be due to a rise in blood-pressure or other problems. If you have suddenly started to get headaches, consult your doctor.

RIGHT **Avoid alcohol, dairy products, citrus fruit, chocolate and caffeine if you suffer from migraines.**

COFFEE

ALCOHOL

CHOCOLATE

CHEESE

CITRUS FRUIT

GENERAL
ACHING

DISTENDING
OR THROBBING
PAIN

HEAVY, DULL,
NAGGING
ACHE

RIGHT **Massage throbbing temples with small, circular movements to help alleviate the pain.**

Types of headache

FOREHEAD

This area is controlled by the Stomach and Large Intestine Channels.

Pain: Dull, aching or heavy.

Causes: Qi Deficiency (the pain will be brought on by tiredness or lack of food). Dampness (the pain will be worse in the mornings and will affect the concentration, with a muzzy sensation). In practice, the two syndromes are often combined.

Herbs: Modified Clear the Spleen decoction (omit Lian Zi and Yi Zhi Ren, add Ju Hua and Yan Hu Suo).

Avoid: Irregular meals and insufficient rest (these cause Qi Deficiency); dairy produce, bread, yeast and sugar (prone to cause Dampness).

BASE OF SKULL

Pain: Dull and aching, worse when tired or after a period.

Causes: Chronic (long-term) pain at the back of the head is due to Blood Deficiency of the Liver and Kidneys. Acute (sudden) pain in this area will often be caused by a cold or flu, when there will be tightness and a stiff neck.

Herbs: Modified Strengthen the Kidney decoction (increase dose of Chuan Xiong by half).

Avoid: Alcohol, caffeine.

TOP OF HEAD

Pain: Dull, empty sensation. May be accompanied by dizziness and is better when lying down.

Causes: Liver Blood Deficiency, in which case the eyes will also often be dry or gritty.

Herbs: Modified Nourish the Blood decoction (increase dose of Gou Qi Zi by half).

Avoid: Alcohol, caffeine.

TEMPLES/BEHIND THE EYES/
SIDES OF HEAD/ONE-SIDED

Pain: These areas are commonly associated with migraines and pain is usually throbbing or distending in nature.

Causes: Liver energy surging upwards to the head.

Herbs: Modified Free the Liver decoction (add Yan Hu Suo and Mu Dan Pi, reduce dose of Chai Hu by half).

Avoid: Migraine triggers such as alcohol, dairy products, caffeine, citrus fruits and chocolate. As stress is also a factor, relaxation and meditation techniques will be helpful.

ALLERGIES

敏感

ABOVE **One of the Chinese characters for an allergic syndrome.**

The rise in the numbers of people complaining of allergic conditions has multiplied by an astonishing amount over the last decade. Some of these are well documented, such as asthma and hay fever. Others are new phenomena which have divided medical opinion as to whether their cause is physical or psychosomatic (in the mind). This second group includes problems such as extreme food allergies, candidiasis (yeast overgrowth) and chemical sensitivity.

Fighting the problem

Conventional medicine has been slow to provide satisfactory remedies, so many people have been forced to turn to non-conventional therapies for relief.

Many allergic reactions are the result of the body's immune system responding to a stress, such as hay fever being caused by pollen. Allergies are also commonly involved in the modern problem of chronic fatigue immuno-deficiency syndromes (CFIDS).

Many people find ways of living with their problem by avoiding the allergen, but some people can be so sensitive that almost anything can trigger a reaction, and these are the people who may have to alter their lifestyles drastically in order to survive.

BELOW **It's hard to escape from allergens – they are everywhere.**

ASSAULT ON THE IMMUNE SYSTEM

There are many reasons for this sudden rise in allergies (even asthma was regarded as a rare disease until recently). They include an increased level of toxins in the environment from pollution, chemical fertilizers, household products, and contaminated water. Other contributory factors are the routine use of antibiotics, which depletes the immune system, and the poor-quality diet that many people eat.

Interestingly, in Chinese Medicine there is no single word for allergy. The immune system is not viewed as a solitary concept, but is considered to be made up of a number of different systems with separate functions. There are several Chinese words that express the idea of immune reaction, and these usually crop up in allergies and sensitivities.

Types of allergy and sensitivity

敏感

- Asthma
- Rheumatoid arthritis
- Hay fever
- Food intolerance or sensitivity

- Chronic candidiasis
- Multiple chemical sensitivity
- House-dust mites, dust, animals, pollution

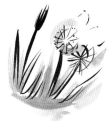

POLLEN

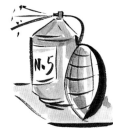

DUST MITES

PERFUME

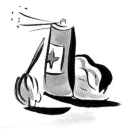

HOUSEHOLD PRODUCTS

CROSS CHECK Damp, Phlegm and Food Stagnation *pages 42–45,*
Detoxification *pages 94–95*

THE CHINESE THREE-STEP PLAN

In Chinese Medicine, there is no distinction between mind and body, so that which affects the body will affect the mind, and vice versa. To tackle an allergy, a three-step approach is followed.

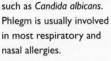

| Identify and remove the offending substances.

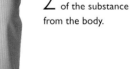

2 Clear the build-up of the substance from the body.

3 Identify and correct the Deficiency that is allowing the reaction to occur.

Chinese concepts of allergies

While Traditional Chinese Medicine has little concept of the allergies that preoccupy many Western sufferers, the symptoms associated with allergies are defined in classic terms: assault by the various Evils, an imbalance of Fluids leading to Dampness or Phlegm, or some sort of weakness (Deficiency) in the affected organs.

WIND

Wind is one of the external Evils. The Chinese character for Wind is an insect being borne through the air. Wind expresses the idea of something malevolent being carried into the body via the nose or mouth. Wind can also be retained in the body, causing overreactions.

DAMPNESS AND PHLEGM

Dampness correlates with the idea of fungal infections that provide an ideal breeding ground for yeasts such as *Candida albicans*. Phlegm is usually involved in most respiratory and nasal allergies.

POISON

Toxins can be retained or generated in the body, and a build-up will cause the immune system to over-react to any additional workload, causing the familiar allergic response of inflammation and mucus.

DEFICIENCY

Deficiency of the Qi, Blood or functioning of the internal organs, is almost always combined with the presence of one or more of the above, and it is this that makes allergies so hard to treat. In most cases, it is not enough to simply remove the offending substance: unless the Deficiency is also rectified, the person will remain sensitive to the substance and will probably develop new reactions as well.

The three-step approach is a complex process that really requires the assistance of a properly qualified Chinese Medicine physician, but here is a very basic three-step plan you can try for yourself.

🐾 Eliminate the problem substances from your life. The foods that most commonly cause allergic reactions are dairy products, yeast, bread, sugar, citrus and tropical fruits, chemical preservatives, colourings, flavourings, coffee and alcohol.

🐾 Cleanse the body by following the detoxification guidelines on *pages 94–95.*

🐾 Strengthen the body: eat regularly and properly, get at least eight hours' sleep, and exercise or meditate to help cope with stress.

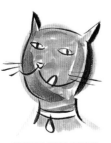

PETS AND OTHER ANIMALS

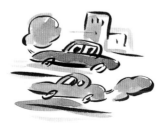

POLLUTION

WOMEN'S HEALTH

The female anatomy and physiology is considerably more complex than the male. There are a number of specific issues that women have to deal with in life: menstruation, pregnancy and menopause. It is important to remind ourselves that none of these is a disease. All three are normal physiological processes, which most women will go through without problems. The common element in all three areas is the Chinese concept of the Blood, which is the basis of the saying 'Women's lives are dominated by Blood.'

ABOVE **Chinese Medicine divides a woman's life into three stages: puberty, fertility and menopause.**

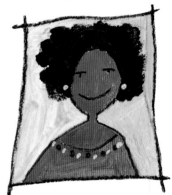

ABOVE **According to Chinese Medicine, menstruation should be free from pain and emotional upset.**

Menstruation

The Chinese approach to period problems relies on comparisons with what is termed a 'normal' period. Normal periods should start between the ages of twelve and fourteen, arrive every 28 days, and last for around five days. There should be a moderate amount of bleeding which is neither scanty nor flooding, and the blood should be fresh and without clots. There should be no pain, and no dramatic fluctuations in mood.

This may confuse women who have been told by a doctor that the problems they have with their periods are 'normal' – these should more accurately be described as common problems.

By treating period problems early, more problematic health issues can be avoided in later life. The nature of your periods is a good gauge to your general health, and you can use this to correct potential imbalances before they happen.

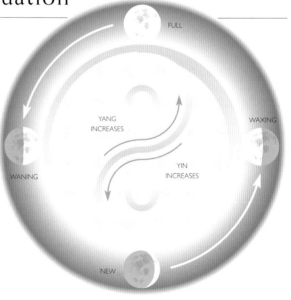

ABOVE **Yin and Yang increase and decrease with the lunar cycle.**

Menstrual problems

IRREGULAR PERIODS

Symptoms: A cycle which fluctuates by more than a week under or over the usual length of four weeks.

Cause: Kidney and Liver Deficiency.

Tongue: Pale.

Pulse: Empty.

Herbs: Nourish the Blood decoction.

PAINFUL PERIODS

Symptoms: Pain before and during the period.

Cause: Qi and Blood Stasis.

Tongue: Variable.

Pulse: Full if there is pain.

Herbs: Regulate the Blood decoction.

Symptoms: Pain after the period has stopped.

Cause: Blood Deficiency.

Herbs: Nourish the Blood decoction.

NO PERIODS

For periods stopping after a normal cycle has been established

Symptoms: Periods become lighter and then stop.

Cause: Blood Deficiency

Tongue: Pale.

Pulse: Empty.

Herbs: Nourish the Blood decoction.

Symptoms: Periods are painful, with clots, and then stop.

Cause: Blood Stagnation.

Tongue: Variable.

Pulse: Full.

Herbs: Regulate the Blood decoction.

For periods not starting at all

Symptoms: Periods have not started by the age of fifteen.

Cause: Kidney Deficiency.

Herbs: Strengthen the Kidney decoction.

PRE-MENSTRUAL SYNDROME (PMS)

Symptoms: Mood swings, irritability, depression, breast pain, carbohydrate and sugar cravings, changes to bowel habits, outbreaks of acne.

Cause: Liver Stagnation and Blood Deficiency.

Tongue: Pale or mauve.

Pulse: Empty after period, Full beforehand.

Herbs: Free the Liver decoction.

DYSFUNCTIONAL BLEEDING

There are a number of causes of bleeding outside the normal cycle, or periods that arrive more frequently than every month, or that last more than a week. They are too complex to describe within the scope of this book, and some of the patterns represent potentially serious conditions which are best treated by a doctor or trained physician.

STANDING POLE POSITION

POSTURE IS HELD FOR TWO MINUTES

RIGHT **Qi Gong helps to strengthen the body and relax the mind: beneficial at any time of life.**

ESSENTIALS
Menstrual problems are closely related to Liver disharmonies.

Blood Deficiency can lead to imbalance, which often causes period problems.

Pregnancy

Look after yourself by eating properly, getting enough sleep (while you can) and avoiding physical and mental stress. Chinese Medicine sees a direct link between the emotional state of a mother and the health of her baby, so a wise woman will endeavour to keep herself apart from stressful situations at work and at home.

During pregnancy, women enter a much more internal world. The pulse is nearly always Slippery – this is normal and reflects the additional fluids in the body. The appearance of the tongue will vary according to the woman's general constitution.

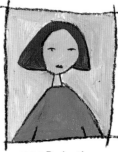

ABOVE **During the childbearing years, the health of the Blood is especially important.**

AVOID MENTAL STRESS

GET PLENTY OF REST

EAT A NUTRITIOUS, WELL-BALANCED DIET

MAINTAIN A PROGRAMME OF GENTLE EXERCISE

Ginger tea

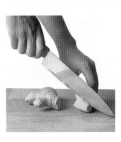

1 Ginger tea helps fight nausea. Peel a small chunk of fresh ginger root, and cut into 3–6 slices.

2 Put the sliced ginger into a saucepan with some water, and simmer for 3–5 minutes.

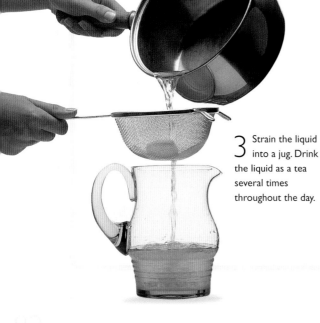

3 Strain the liquid into a jug. Drink the liquid as a tea several times throughout the day.

CAUTION

Particular care must be taken when self-medicating during pregnancy. It is best to consult a doctor before taking any herbs.

ABOVE **To ensure a baby's pre-natal Qi is good, a woman must take good care of herself during her pregnancy.**

Common conditions during and after pregnancy

MORNING SICKNESS

Fresh ginger root (Sheng Jiang) will do much to remedy morning sickness. Try making your own ginger tea, or buy ginger tea bags. Even ginger beer can be of some benefit. If this doesn't do the trick, Xiang Sha Liu Jun Zi Wan is a safe remedy, available in pill form. Take 4–8 of the small black pills twice to three times daily.

BACK PAIN

There are obvious physical reasons for the back being under strain during pregnancy. However, ensuring you get enough rest will help, as will yoga or Tai Qi. Women who do these forms of exercise also tend to have easier births.

If your back is weak and always sore, with very frequent urination, try a Strengthen the Kidney decoction.

HIGH BLOOD-PRESSURE AND WATER RETENTION

If your blood-pressure rises during pregnancy (particularly if this is accompanied by fluid retention and protein in the urine), your doctor will monitor you closely.

However, there are things you can do. A nutritious diet will help prevent the advent of symptoms, and may control them if they start. Never restrict your calorie intake during pregnancy: aim for no less than 2800 calories a day. Most women will benefit from a magnesium and calcium supplement (ratio 2:1). Try replacing table salt with kelp flakes (Kun Bu) on your food.

If, in spite of all these measures, you develop hypertension and oedema, try a herbal tincture of juniper berry, nettle leaf, celery seed, or parsley (in last week of pregnancy only, as this herb stimulates the uterus).

THREATENED MISCARRIAGE

Always consult your doctor if you get any spotting during pregnancy. Most of the time it does not pose an immediate threat, but if you are concerned or have a history of miscarriage, lie down and stay there. If necessary you should not balk at lying down for the whole of the last few weeks of your pregnancy.

STRETCH MARKS

Massaging oils into the abdomen and perineum regularly during pregnancy and after labour will help to repair stretch marks. Use sesame oil (Hei Zhi Ma) as a base, and add a few drops of the essential oils of borage or evening primrose, vitamin E, carrot, and rose.

For a herbal remedy, try a Strengthen the Blood decoction.

ESSENTIALS

A baby's parental Qi levels depend on the mother's health.

Seek professional help quickly for any persistent symptoms during pregnancy.

POSTNATAL DEPRESSION

Chinese Medicine considers Blood Deficiency to be one of the main causes of this problem. Even if you have not lost a lot of blood as a result of the birth, remember that you 'donate' a large volume of your blood to your baby, and this can be enough to cause an emotional plunge.

Your own placenta (Zi He Che) is a very rich source of Blood nutrients. If the idea of eating it (cooked like liver or made into a pâté) is unappealing, it can be dried and made into capsules.

Remove the umbilical cord and membrane and wash the placenta in running water for several hours. Slice it thinly and place in the oven on the lowest heat for around 15–20 hours, until completely dried out. This can then be powdered in a food processor and put into pill capsules.

KNEAD FIRMLY

FORM A FIST

DEPENDING ON THE PROBLEM, RUB CLOCKWISE OR ANTICLOCKWISE

LEFT **Warm the Kidneys by rubbing your fists either side of the spine at the waist.**

LEFT **Warm the lower abdomen by rubbing it gently clockwise.**

Menopause

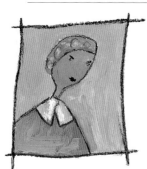

ABOVE **Although some women regret the end of fertility, for others it brings new freedom.**

The menopause is a natural phase for all women. The ending of the monthly period marks the end of fertility, and this gives many women a new lease of life, free from the constraints of contraception and menstruation. For many women, there is a need to find a new 'role' at the menopause. By this time, children may no longer be so dependent on them, and relationships with partners can become strained. For a few, the normal menopause may be disharmonious. Symptoms related to changes in the nature of the Blood, as it is understood in Chinese Medicine, occur. This is a much more common phenomenon in the West; in traditional cultures women have a much smoother transition, with fewer associated symptoms such as hot flushes, night sweats, mood swings and anxiety.

AGEING GRACEFULLY?

There are several reasons for this difference between cultures. Not least amongst them are the social constraints placed on women in the West. An obsession with youth, and fixed ideas of what constitutes beauty, tend to lead to an undervaluing of 'older' women in society. This loss of status leads many women to resort to chemical hormonal supplementation to slow down the natural ageing process.

For some women, hormone replacement therapy can lead to a dramatic alleviation of menopausal symptoms; many other people find they are unable to tolerate the drugs and develop side-effects that force them to stop. In either case, the potential benefits of HRT need to be weighed up against the potential long-term effects, which include a higher incidence of certain forms of cancer.

NATURAL PROGRESSION

In Traditional Chinese Medicine a woman's life is counted in periods of seven years – menstruation is expected to start at fourteen and end at 49, although most women will not conform to this neat model. The menopause is associated with a gradual and quite natural depletion of Kidney essence (Jing), which is closely linked with inherited Qi. As we grow older, Kidney weakness can clearly be seen in the senses and tissues related to the Kidneys: our hair turns grey and there may eventually be hearing loss. This Kidney weakness can help explain some of the common menopausal problems. The

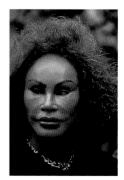

LEFT **Pressure to remain forever young is an increasing burden for Western women, leading many to resort to cosmetic surgery, which may not always be an unqualified success.**

Kidneys are linked to the Water Element, and so can lead to a flaring of Fire with irritability, sweating, hot flushes and dizziness. General weakness in Kidney Yin and Yang can be seen in back pain, alternating bouts of feeling hot and cold, dizziness and tinnitus. Associated Excess Liver Fire can lead to angry outbursts and emotional distress. Chinese herbal remedies used for menopausal problems often include herbs for strengthening the Kidneys, such as He Shou Wu or Nu Zhen Zi.

ESSENTIALS
Menopausal ailments may be due to a gradual depletion of Qi or Blood.

With a healthy diet and lifestyle, many women will find the menopause brings few health problems.

LEFT **Remaining active and receptive to new ideas and experiences ensures life remains challenging and interesting.**

HELPING YOURSELF

If you are worried about approaching menopause, or are experiencing symptoms already, there are many things you can do to protect yourself naturally without resorting to drugs. As these treatments are gentle, try following the advice given here to begin with. You still have the option of trying HRT at a later stage if you find that the effects are insufficient for your purposes.

FOOD

Make sure you are getting proper nutrition. The ideal diet will accentuate grain and vegetables, fish and fresh fruit. You need to be getting enough minerals and protein, without eating too many heavy foods or relying on dairy produce and meat. Coffee (including decaffeinated) has a dramatic effect on destabilizing the hormones and is best avoided completely. Substitute herbal teas instead, and drink plenty of water.

VALUABLE OILS

Oily fish are important sources of nutrition, particularly salmon, mackerel, herring and tuna. They are rich in omega-3 and omega-6 essential fatty acids. These may also be found in olive and sesame oils, but particularly in flax (linseed) and hemp oils, both of which are becoming increasingly available through healthfood stores. Aim to have around three tablespoons of one or a mixture of these oils daily. They can be used as dressings, served with vegetables, included in many dishes, or taken in juice.

BOOSTER FOODS

Calcium is an important mineral for preserving the health of the bones and preventing osteoporosis. Find it in milk, cheese, eggs, salmon, leafy green vegetables, soy beans, beans and nuts. Sesame is an especially rich source of calcium and is found in humous or tahini (sesame and chickpea paste). Two other weapons against osteoporosis are vitamin D and magnesium. Vitamin D is found in milk, eggs, oily fish, cheese and cod-liver oil. It is also derived from exposure to sunlight. Magnesium sources include soy beans, nuts and brewer's yeast.

One of the health secrets of oriental women is tofu, a solid curd made from soy beans. Tofu should be bought fresh (preferably organic) and can be used as it is, or marinated and added to stirfries, roasts, grills or soups. Tofu has particular health benefits for women and regular consumption seems to offer protection against a range of diseases.

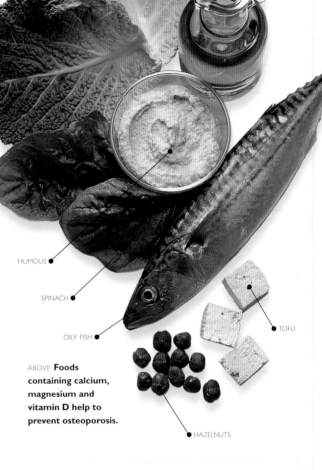

CABBAGE

LINSEED OIL

HUMOUS

SPINACH

OILY FISH

TOFU

HAZELNUTS

ABOVE **Foods containing calcium, magnesium and vitamin D help to prevent osteoporosis.**

Menopausal disharmonies

HOT-TYPE MENOPAUSE

Symptoms: Marked hot flushes or night sweats, anxiety, poor concentration and short-term memory, loss of confidence, insomnia, low backache, vaginal dryness, dry-type constipation.

Herbs: Nourish the Kidney decoction.

COLD-TYPE MENOPAUSE

Symptoms: Mild flushes, depression, weight gain, water retention and oedema, poor concentration and short-term memory, loss of confidence, back pain, tiredness, and loose stools.

Herbs: Strengthen the Kidney decoction.

MEN'S HEALTH

BELOW **As for women, Chinese Medicine divides a man's life into a series of stages.**

In Traditional Chinese Medicine a man's life is counted in stages of eight years, with puberty at sixteen. This section looks at health problems solely encountered by men – largely problems associated with the male reproductive system and urinary disorders. It does not cover problems men and women are equally likely to suffer.

The genitourinary system

Although men suffer from cystitis (inflammation of the bladder) less frequently than women – largely because a man's urethra (which connects the bladder to the outside world) is longer than a woman's – they can be prone to other urinary tract disorders and may have problems connected with urinary flow. Difficulty in urinating is very common in men over 50. The prostate gland is commonly associated with these problems. Indeed, it seems probable that almost all men will have some enlargement of the prostate in later life, but in the great majority of cases this will be benign (non-cancerous).

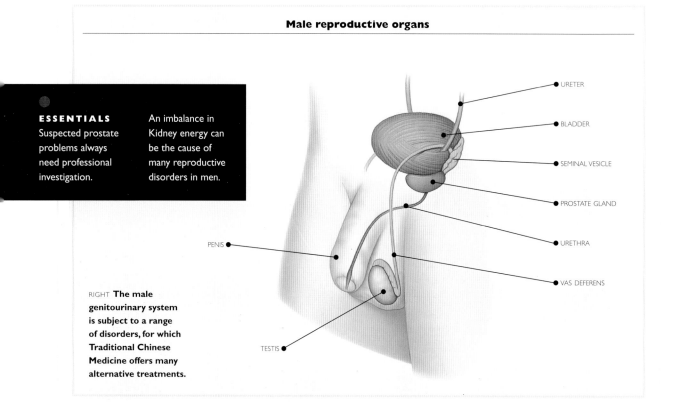

Male reproductive organs

ESSENTIALS
Suspected prostate problems always need professional investigation.

An imbalance in Kidney energy can be the cause of many reproductive disorders in men.

URETER

BLADDER

SEMINAL VESICLE

PROSTATE GLAND

URETHRA

VAS DEFERENS

PENIS

TESTIS

RIGHT **The male genitourinary system is subject to a range of disorders, for which Traditional Chinese Medicine offers many alternative treatments.**

Male disharmonies

URINARY PROBLEMS

General difficulty with urination, which may be slow to start, or have interrupted flow. There may be dribbling and frequent urination, severe lower abdominal pain and backache.

Burning pain

Symptoms: As above plus burning and strong pain on urination; dark, cloudy, strong-smelling urine; fever, high thirst.

Tongue: May be red.

Pulse: Rapid, Full.

Herbs: Clear the Bladder decoction.

Mild discomfort

Symptoms: Mild pain or discomfort on urination, feeling hot in the evening.

Tongue: Red, peeled patches.

Pulse: Rapid.

Herbs: Nourish the Kidney decoction.

Extreme frequency

Symptoms: Very frequent urination, tiredness or exhaustion, feeling cold, heaviness in the abdomen, no pain.

Tongue: Pale, swollen.

Pulse: Empty, Deep.

Herbs: Strengthen the Kidney decoction.

Frequency

Symptoms: Frequent passing of cloudy, pale urine, heaviness in the abdomen, tiredness, no pain.

Tongue: Sticky coating.

Pulse: Full.

Herbs: Drain the Bladder decoction.

SEXUAL PROBLEMS

Three common problems are lack of erection, low sperm count and poor sperm quality.

Erectile difficulties

Symptoms: Inability to get or sustain an erection, low backache, insomnia, feeling hot in the evening, thirst, and constipation.

Tongue: Red, peeled patches.

Pulse: Rapid, can be Full or Empty.

Herbs: Nourish the Kidney decoction.

Symptoms: Inability to get or sustain an erection, weak and painful back and knees, feeling the cold, loose stools or diarrhoea.

Tongue: Pale.

Pulse: Deep, Empty.

Herbs: Strengthen the Kidney decoction.

Symptoms: Inability to get or sustain an erection, weakness and heaviness in the legs, concentrated urine. The condition is due to descending Damp-Heat.

Tongue: Slimy, yellow coating.

Pulse: Deep, Slippery, Rapid.

Reproductive problems

Symptoms: Low sperm count, poor sperm quality or motility, low back pain and weak knees, feelings of cold, frequent urination, especially at night.

Herbs: Strengthen the Kidney decoction with the addition of Ren Shen and Wu Wei Zi.

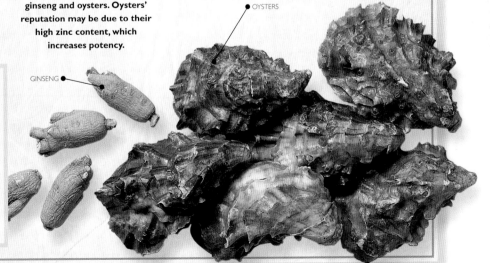

BELOW **Traditional aphrodisiacs: ginseng and oysters. Oysters' reputation may be due to their high zinc content, which increases potency.**

OYSTERS

GINSENG

CAUTION

If a problem persists, or there is pain associated with your symptoms, you should see a doctor to rule out the possibility of a more serious condition.

BABIES AND CHILDREN

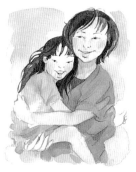

ABOVE **Add fruit juice to herbs if your child finds them unpalatable; do not use sweeteners.**

When treating babies and young children, it is essential to use simple, safe formulas at low dosages. Children under the age of seven are considered to have undeveloped Qi and organ functions. Their condition can change rapidly and fluctuate accordingly. The pulse and tongue are particularly hard to gauge in young children. Chinese physicians usually inspect the index finger, looking at colour and the quality of the blood vessels. This takes skill and practice, so it is best for non-professionals to rely on other symptoms to make a diagnosis.

Diet

RIGHT **Guide your child towards a balanced diet including plenty of fruit and vegetables, to keep him or her in good health.**

Most problems can be traced to diet or digestive function, so to keep your child in good health, make sure that he or she eats properly, and doesn't fill up on sweets and snacks.

The traditional Chinese view of what to feed babies and young children is quite different from that in the West. At a young age, the digestive system is said to be very immature, so children will find it hard to digest or absorb heavy foods.

It is very easy for children to develop conditions linked to the concepts of Phlegm and Dampness, such as colic, glue ear, coughs, asthma, sleeping difficulties, diarrhoea, and difficult behaviour. If we take a look at the foods commonly given to children in the West, we can see that they are particularly likely to cause the formation of Phlegm and Damp: cow's milk, yoghurt, orange juice, pasta, bananas, sweets, biscuits, crisps, chips, food colourings and E numbers, and hidden sugars in baby foods and products such as baked beans. The artificial ingredients and sugars may also cause behavioural problems. These foods can affect Liver energy, leading to overexuberance of Qi and signs of hyperactivity.

ESSENTIALS
Diet is very important: inappropriate foods can lead to Damp and Phlegm.

—

Diagnosis can be difficult. Consult a professional for any severe or persistent symptoms.

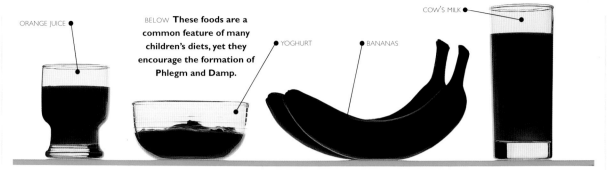

ORANGE JUICE

BELOW **These foods are a common feature of many children's diets, yet they encourage the formation of Phlegm and Damp.**

YOGHURT

BANANAS

COW'S MILK

Childhood illnesses

It can be particularly hard to give young children strange-tasting herbal teas, so you can dilute the appropriate dose in milk or apple juice if required.

Symptoms: A tendency to produce a lot of catarrh, coughing when lying down, ear problems, poor digestion and appetite.

Herbs: Aid the Young Digestion decoction.

Symptoms: Always catching colds, lots of sore throats and swollen glands, tiredness, poor appetite and digestion.

Herbs: Strengthen the Qi in the Young decoction.

WHAT SHOULD I GIVE MY CHILD?

Children need a simple and bland diet. This can be very hard to maintain as it requires more effort on the part of the parents, and necessitates proper supervision at nurseries and when offspring are to be fed by other people. However, it is much easier to start by feeding your children in this way, rather than to try and cut out foods once they have a taste for them.

BABIES UNDER 1 YEAR

Breastfeeding meets all nutritional requirements at this age. If you are unable to breastfeed, use goat's or sheep's milk, which is much closer to human milk than cow's milk. Milk can be supplemented with rice porridge if your baby is hungry and the milk is not enough to keep her happy.

AGE 1–3

Introduce cooked vegetables such as steamed, mashed or baked carrots, parsnips, broccoli, cauliflower, and potatoes. Carbohydrates should come mostly from grains such as rice and barley, rather than a lot of bread and wheat pasta. The child will enjoy fruit such as apples and pears. For an alternative dessert, give goat's or sheep's yoghurt. Diluted pure apple or pear juice is popular. In general, children of this age don't really need any meat or fish.

AGE 3 ONWARDS

Slowly introduce different foods, in more complex combinations, and use different ways of cooking. Fish and meat can be given as required.

Herb dosages for children

shown as proportion of adult dose

- Under 6 months: ⅙ dose.
- 6–12 months: ⅛ dose.
- 12–24 months: ¼ dose.
- 2–4 years: ⅓ dose.
- 4–7 years: ½ dose.
- 7–14 years: ⅔ dose.
- 14 and above: give the adult dose.

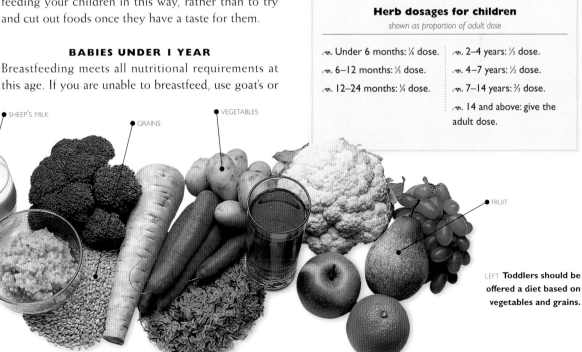

SHEEP'S MILK

GRAINS

VEGETABLES

FRUIT

LEFT **Toddlers should be offered a diet based on vegetables and grains.**

89

EMOTIONAL ISSUES

Think about the stresses of our modern world. Most of us don't have to worry too much about physical concerns such as keeping warm, or having a roof over our heads. Instead we are weighed down by relationship difficulties, financial concerns, and job insecurity. These types of stress partly explain the much higher incidence of mental and emotional problems found in industrialized countries, compared to traditional cultures.

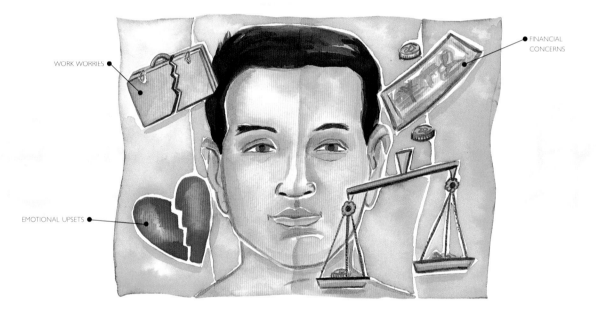

WORK WORRIES

FINANCIAL CONCERNS

EMOTIONAL UPSETS

Mind and body

Today there is much talk of holism and the intimate connection between the mind-body-spirit, but to a Chinese doctor, saying that the mind affects the body is stating the obvious.

ABOVE **Broken relationships, job insecurity, and money worries insidiously affect emotional well-being.**

THE BIG PICTURE

What this means is that physical problems can affect mental state, and emotions can have a bearing on physical health. This can be seen when an organ is out of balance. For example, Spleen Qi Deficiency can lead to tiredness, diarrhoea, poor concentration and a tendency to worry. The Five Elements also illustrate this particularly clearly, as they are physical-emotional pictures of body types. Looking at the information for, say, the Wood type, you will discover that there may be anger and irritability as well as problems such as period pain, or poor eyesight. By working out the correct pattern or body type, any physical, mental or emotional problems present can be alleviated together.

INSOMNIA

The Heart is the seat of individual consciousness, giving us the ability to be calm and therefore to sleep soundly. The Chinese concept of Heart problems should not be confused with the idea of heart disease in conventional medicine: having a 'Heart' disharmony does not mean that you are going to have a heart attack! The Heart is often involved in insomnia, which is likely to result from the presence of Heat, producing hyperactivity, or a Deficiency. Other triggers are a lack of Blood, causing the Mind to wander, or a disharmonious Liver, leading to restlessness. Identifying the exact cause is important in order to select an appropriate remedy.

ESSENTIALS
Life in modern Western society is far more stressful than life in ancient China, but the way the emotions relate to organs continues to be relevant, as is taking a holistic approach to health.

LEFT **Restless nights may be attributed to problems with the Heart, Liver, Blood or Yin.**

Insomnia problems

HEART DEFICIENCY

Symptoms: Palpitations, tiredness, shortness of breath on exertion, pale sallow complexion, insomnia, excess dreaming, anxiety.

Tongue: Pale, thin, may have a crack in the tip.

Pulse: Empty.

Herbs: Nourish the Heart decoction.

HEART HEAT

Symptoms: Palpitations, agitation, anxiety, insomnia, red complexion or cheeks, dark urine, thirst, and mouth or tongue ulcers.

Tongue: Red tip, possibly with central crack to tip.

Pulse: May be Full or Empty (depending on severity), or Rapid.

Herbs: Nourish and Calm the Heart decoction.

BLOOD DEFICIENCY

Symptoms: Waking suddenly, vivid dreams, anxiety, dry skin and hair, tiredness, light periods, dry-type constipation.

Tongue: Pale, dry.

Pulse: Empty.

Herbs: Nourish the Blood decoction.

LIVER STAGNATION

Symptoms: Mind too active to go to sleep, irritability and mood swings, dream-disturbed sleep, anxiety attacks, or depression.

Tongue: Mauve or purple.

Pulse: Full.

Herbs: Modified Free the Liver decoction (add Suan Zao Ren).

YIN DEFICIENCY

Symptoms: Difficulty in falling or staying asleep, feeling hot at night and night sweats, low backache, a need to urinate during the night, thirst, constipation.

Tongue: Red, peeled patches.

Pulse: Can be Full or Empty, Superficial.

Herbs: Nourish the Kidney decoction.

ANXIETY AND PANIC ATTACKS

The pace at which most of us lead our lives hardly leaves pause for breath. Activity levels like these, at the expense of proper rest, give rise to feelings of anxiety and panic. It is important to remember how these emotional upsets can affect the body's organs, upsetting the Yin-Yang balance or depleting the Qi and Blood. The consumption of stimulants (coffee, alcohol, tobacco, illegal drugs) leads to Heat, causing hyperactivity. If you have trouble sleeping, are anxious, or if you are regularly aware of your heart beating, cut down your intake of stimulants. It is important to do this gradually, to allow your mind and body time to adjust. Ensure you get enough rest.

IN AN EMERGENCY

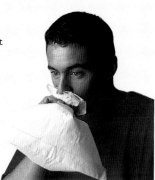

Hyperventilation can cause symptoms such as breathlessness, a tight chest and feelings of panic. If this happens, breathe in and out of a paper bag for a few minutes to alter your carbon dioxide levels, and you will quickly feel better.

Breathing exercise

One of the best ways of controlling anxiety and helping relaxation is to do simple breathing exercises. Most people don't know how to breathe properly.

STAGE ONE

DIAPHRAGM BREATHING

- Lie down on a firm surface or sit in a straight-backed chair and relax.
- Put one hand on the centre of your chest, the other one over your belly button, and become aware of how you are breathing.
- If you are moving the upper part of your ribcage rather than your abdomen, then you may be hyperventilating. Practise breathing using the abdomen, by making sure the hand on your chest doesn't move, and with the hand on your tummy rising and falling as you breathe in and out.
- Count as you breathe – count to four as you breathe in, and again as you breathe out.

STAGE TWO

FOUR-CYCLE BREATHING

After you have practised diaphragm breathing for a while, go on to this.

- Count to four as you breathe in, then pause for a count of four.
- Breathe out as you count to four, then pause for a count of four.

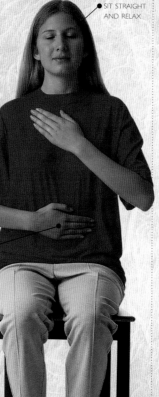

SIT STRAIGHT AND RELAX

ABDOMEN SHOULD RISE AND FALL WITH EACH BREATH

RIGHT **Diaphragm breathing helps relaxation. Start by assessing the quality of your breathing.**

STAGE THREE

RELAXING WHILE BREATHING OUT

You only need to contract muscles when breathing in, not out.

- Practise relaxing as you breathe out, releasing all muscle tension. This will be facilitated by making a gentle 'hmmmmh' noise at the end of the out-breath.
- Work at a natural, slow breathing rhythm. Aim to get your breathing down to about six to eight cycles per minute (this will take time).
- When you feel comfortable with this exercise, start to incorporate your relaxation practice into gentle everyday activities such as walking, doing chores, and shopping.
- With practice you will start to breathe in a more natural way. Around twenty minutes' practice a day is ideal.

BELOW **Breathing exercises can be fitted into the working day.**

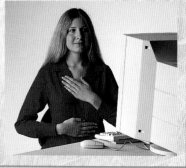

Anxiety problems

HEART DEFICIENCY

Symptoms: Anxiety, palpitations, tiredness, shortness of breath on exertion, pale sallow complexion, insomnia, excessive dreaming, anxiety.

Tongue: Pale, thin, may have a crack in the tip.

Pulse: Empty.

Herbs: Nourish the Heart decoction.

HEART HEAT

Symptoms: Palpitations, agitation, anxiety, insomnia, red complexion or red cheeks, dark urine, thirst, mouth or tongue ulcers.

Tongue: Red tip, possibly with central crack to tip.

Pulse: May be Full or Empty (depending on severity), Rapid.

Herbs: Nourish and Calm the Heart decoction.

BLOOD DEFICIENCY

Symptoms: Waking suddenly, vivid dreams, anxiety, dry skin and hair, tiredness, light periods, and dry-type constipation.

Tongue: Pale, dry.

Pulse: Empty.

Herbs: Nourish the Blood decoction.

LIVER STAGNATION

Symptoms: Mind too active to go to sleep, irritability and mood swings, dream-disturbed sleep, anxiety or depression.

Tongue: Mauve or purple.

Pulse: Full.

Herbs: Modified Free the Liver decoction (add Suan Zao Ren).

YIN DEFICIENCY

Symptoms: Difficulty in falling or staying asleep, anxiety, feeling hot at night and night sweats, low backache, a need to urinate during the night, thirst, constipation.

Tongue: Red, peeled patches.

Pulse: Can be Full or Empty, Superficial.

Herbs: Nourish the Kidney decoction.

BELOW **The five emotions (fear, excessive joy, anger, grief and worry) can cause ill-health. Depression may follow on from any of these.**

ESSENTIALS
Stress and anxiety can interfere with Qi and Blood, and lead to imbalances.

The five emotions can have a detrimental effect on the body's organs, leading to ill-health.

Depression problems

Depression can be the main cause of disharmony, or it can come about as the result of another illness. There is massive variation in what people mean when they say they are depressed – it can vary from feeling low to clinical depression, where life is dominated by feelings of blackness. People with severe depression may well be taking conventionally prescribed drugs, and care should be taken to consult a doctor to ensure there will be no clash between the drugs and herbs.

LIVER STAGNATION

Symptoms: Depression, anger, irritability, frustration, PMS, distending sensation on the flanks, restless sleep.

Tongue: Purple or mauve.

Pulse: Full.

Herbs: Modified Free the Liver decoction (add Yu Jin). If there is also a bitter taste in mouth, indigestion and constipation, add Mu Dan Pi and Huang Lian.

YANG DEFICIENCY

Symptoms: Depression, tiredness and lethargy, weakness, feeling cold, backache, frequent urination.

Tongue: Pale and swollen.

Pulse: Empty and Deep.

Herbs: Modified Strengthen the Kidney decoction (add Yu Jin and Chai Hu).

SPLEEN DEFICIENCY WITH DAMPNESS

Symptoms: Tiredness and lethargy, muscle aches, depression, poor concentration and memory, lack of appetite, loose stools or diarrhoea, dull headaches.

Tongue: Pale, swollen, sticky coating.

Pulse: Can be Empty or Full.

Herbs: Modified Clear the Spleen decoction (add Yu Jin and Chai Hu).

DETOXIFICATION

Detoxification programmes are for healthy people with a robust digestion, who want to clear the body of accumulated toxins. It is common to have some withdrawal symptoms when following a programme of this nature, but if these are strong, then you have probably tried to do too much too soon. Detoxification is an activity that is appropriate for spring and summer, rather than autumn or winter.

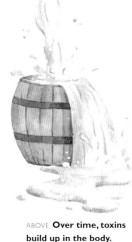

ABOVE **Over time, toxins build up in the body. Dedicating a short period to flushing them out is very effective.**

The programme

The most common reaction to the detoxification food plan is to think that there are no 'normal' foods left for you to live on. We all forget that it is our diet in the West that is abnormal. Most of the world's population has lived happily and healthily for the last few thousand years on a diet similar to the one that follows.

RIGHT **On a detoxification programme, you need to monitor the foods you put into your body and follow simple rules about the way you eat.**

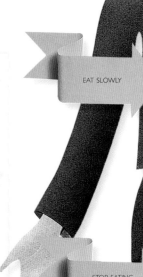

EAT SITTING AT A TABLE

EAT SLOWLY

STOP EATING BEFORE YOU ARE FULL

Food you cannot eat

Foods to stop entirely for a period of four weeks:

- All products containing yeast. Unleavened 'flat' breads without yeast, such as pitta, are okay.

- Wheat products. Products such as multi-grain bread, with a maximum wheatflour content of 50%, are okay.

- All sugars and sweeteners (this also includes honey).

- All dairy products (including soy milk).

- All fruit, dried fruit and fruit juice apart from lemons. (This does not apply during fruit fast.)

- Meat.

- Shellfish.

- All alcohol.

- Anything preserved or fermented.

- Foods containing E-numbers, preservatives, colourings; packaged and convenience foods, foods grown with pesticides.

- Pickles, vinegar and mushrooms.

- All food that is not totally fresh or within its sell-by date.

• Caffeine (tea, coffee, chocolate, fizzy drinks).

• Any drugs you can manage without.

Food you can eat

- Vegetables: as much and any type that you want, but no more than half of them should be raw. The way foods are cooked can also affect their quality. Eat freshly prepared food rather than dishes that have been pre-cooked, chilled and then reheated.

- Wholegrains: rice, barley, quinoa, buckwheat, kasha, amaranth and wild rice.

- Pulses, beans, seeds and nuts (not peanuts).

- Fish (not shellfish).

- Oils: olive, sesame, flax, hempseed, walnut.

- Rice or oat milk.

- One or two eggs a week.

EATING HABITS

How you eat is as important as what you eat.

🐾 Eat slowly, chewing each mouthful thoroughly.

🐾 Do not eat while upset, stressed or busy.

🐾 Eat sitting up at a table, and do not slump on a sofa after you have finished your meal.

🐾 Do not drink any cold fluids with food. Drink hot water or green tea if desired.

🐾 Always eat breakfast, a good lunch and a light dinner no later than 8pm.

🐾 Do not drink or eat any chilled foods, or those taken straight from the fridge.

🐾 Eat until you are only two-thirds full. This leaves room for digestion to take place.

REMEMBER

🐾 Store oils and nuts in the fridge. All oils should be organic and cold-pressed.

🐾 Eat a wide range of foods.

🐾 Eat organic food if possible.

🐾 Use good oils in place of butter.

🐾 Do not heat oils above smoking point.

🐾 Lightly cook all foods, except salads.

🐾 Use only genuine organic sea salt.

🐾 Do not use black pepper during cooking, but add it to your food afterwards.

RIGHT **Flaxseed oil encourages healing; garlic is a natural antibiotic.**

OIL

LEFT **As toxins are cleared from the body, you will experience a range of benefits.**

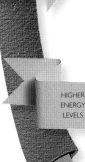

CLEARER SKIN

HIGHER
ENERGY
LEVELS

IMPROVED
DIGESTION

Super foods

ADD THESE TO YOUR DIET

🐾 Flax or hempseed oil. Use in dressings, or in food such as mash. Buy flax (linseed) from a healthfood shop. Do not confuse it with the linseed oil used for DIY!

🐾 Garlic (as much as your family and friends can tolerate).

🐾 Aloe vera (can be made into a drink with water).

🐾 Seaweed (kelp flakes can be sprinkled on food in place of salt).

🐾 Tofu (but not dried soy protein).

🐾 Cayenne pepper (on vegetables, in dressings, soups, stews and mashed potato).

🐾 Liquid aminos in place of soy sauce (buy it from a healthfood shop).

🐾 Ginger or cinnamon (as tea, in stirfries, soups, stews).

🐾 Tahini (sesame paste). Use as peanut butter, in dressings, on baked potatoes.

🐾 Black pepper (uncooked).

🐾 Stevia (a herbal extract) as a sweetener.

🐾 Angostura Bitters. A few drops can be added to water as a refreshing drink. Use 1 teaspoonful in a small glass of water to control sweet cravings.

🐾 Foods to sedate overactive Yang: apples, asparagus, aubergines, barley, celery, cucumber, mushrooms, pears.

🐾 Foods to tonify Yang: radish, raspberries, rice, turnips, leeks, fennel seeds, coriander and cherries.

🐾 Foods that tonify Yin: millet, mulberry, mung beans, duck, oyster, persimmon, pork, tomatoes, and water chestnuts.

GARLIC

GINGER

CINNAMON

TAHINI

SEAWEED

● ESSENTIALS

Specific foods can have a significant effect on your Yin-Yang balance.

—

Detoxification helps to restore harmony and balance, but you need to be in good health: don't do it when recovering from illness.

ABOVE **Ginger is a good source of magnesium. Cinnamon is antibacterial and antifungal. Tahini is rich in essential fatty acids.**

RIGHT **Seaweed is rich in iodine and protein; tofu boasts calcium, magnesium, folic acid and iron.**

TOFU

WHAT DO I EAT FOR BREAKFAST?

Congee, or rice porridge, is the traditional Chinese breakfast. It can be made with any grain, and if you find you are sensitive to rice and barley, you could try quinoa, buckwheat or wild rice. Alternatively, you can use normal oat porridge or sugar-free rice cereal, with rice or oat milk. A small amount of honey (organic cold-pressed) can be added.

FOOD HYGIENE

The mouth is the main route by which pathogens enter the body. All food must be cleaned properly before you eat it. Fruit and vegetables should be soaked and scrubbed in water.

☙ Peel all non-organic fruit and vegetables to help eliminate pesticide residues.

☙ Peel all organic food that is to be eaten raw, in order to get rid of pests.

☙ Soak fish in water, rinse, and cook well.

☙ Salad ingredients should be soaked, rinsed, and any wilted parts discarded.

☙ Do not eat leftovers the next day (soups and stews are acceptable).

☙ Keep a salt shaker of vitamin C powder, and sprinkle on to your food. This is a natural antioxidant.

☙ Avoid eating with your hands whenever possible.

☙ Rinse, in bleach solution, any utensils or kitchen equipment that have been in contact with raw fish.

REHYDRATION

Most people do not drink enough of the right kinds of fluid. Aim to drink around one to three litres of fluids every day. It is wise to 'purge' your tap before refilling filter jugs, by running the water for a minute first. This will get rid of any water that has been contaminated by metals in the piping.

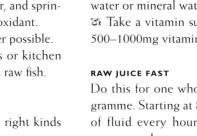

RIGHT **Green tea, herb tea, water, apple juice and carrot juice are suitable for use during a fast.**

RECIPE

CONGEE

*1 part grain
(an espresso cup per person)
4–8 parts water
(depends on how thick
you like your porridge)
3–5 slices fresh ginger
Garnish: seeds, seaweed,
liquid aminos/soy sauce*

Put the grain, water and ginger into a pan. Cook on a very low heat for several hours. Or use an electric slow-cooker, putting it on when you go to bed. You will get up to a ready-made breakfast.

LIQUID AMINOS

SEA

GRAIN

FRESH GINGER

DRINKS AND VITAMINS

The following drinks are the most suitable for drinking during a detoxification programme.

☙ Green or gunpowder tea, single flower or leaf herb teas (or mix herbs to make your own combinations).

☙ Filtered water (change the filter monthly), distilled water or mineral water from glass bottles.

☙ Take a vitamin supplement during detoxification: 500–1000mg vitamin C, two to four times daily.

RAW JUICE FAST

Do this for one whole day in each week of the programme. Starting at 8am, drink a tumbler (300ml/½pt) of fluid every hour until around 8pm, alternating between juice (carrot or apple, the same one all day) and water (see above). Add the juice from a 1cm square piece of fresh ginger to every other glass of juice. Take up to three tablespoonful of hemp, flaxseed, olive or sesame oil three times during the day. Use fresh juice or organic brands. You can eat the same fruit/vegetable as you are drinking; also celery. For dinner, dip celery, apple or carrot into a bowl of oil, with kelp flakes. The day after the fast, eat lightly. Only fast when you are not under pressure. If you have not done it before, do not fast for more than a week. Thereafter, up to a maximum of four weeks is permissible.

CHINESE HERBAL SECRETS

THE HOME MEDICINE CHEST

China is famous for its 'patent' medicines. These traditional, well-known formulas are manufactured under licence in China. Keeping a selection of patent remedies at hand as a herbal medicine chest ensures you are well prepared for treating common ailments quickly and safely.

RIGHT **It is a good idea to keep a stock of the herbs you use most often.**

Colds

Patent remedy: *Gan Mao Ling.*

Only really effective if taken within a day of onset of symptoms.

Colds are probably the most common illness in the world, and yet there is no reliable Western treatment to deal with them. The common symptoms are stiff neck and aching muscles, followed by headache, sneezing, running nose, chilliness, fever and sore throat.

Sinusitis

Patent remedy: *Bi Yan Pian.*

The name of this remedy is literally translated as 'nose inflammation pills'. It can be useful for acute attacks of sinus congestion where there is nasal pain, sneezing, thick yellow-green mucus and itching eyes.

Flu

Patent remedy: *Yin Qiao Jie Du Pian.*

Only really effective if taken within a day of onset of symptoms.

Flu is also very common. The main symptoms are sore throat, swollen glands, feverishness, chills, aching muscles and headache.

Injury, bruising and shock

Patent remedy: *Yunnan Bai Yao.*

Yunnan Bai Yao is reputed to have been responsible for much of the success of the Vietnamese troops during the war with the US. Apparently all soldiers were issued with a bottle of this remedy; the effects of the formula were such that the soldiers returned to the battlefield in a very short period of time.

This remedy can be used for any type of injury, including fractures or severe bruising, and when recovering from operations. Its effectiveness lies in its ability to repair bruising and stop bleeding. It can also be used for any heavy bleeding. Available as a powder or in capsules.

Digestive upsets

Patent remedy: *Huo Xiang Zheng Qi Shui/Ye/Pian* (the last word depends on the type).

Covers symptoms such as nausea, vomiting, headache, loose stools, wind and flu-like feelings. Attacks are often associated with changes in the weather or eating bad food. The remedy is also useful for motion or morning sickness. Available as pills or a liquid. Useful for taking on holiday.

Patent remedy: *China Po Chi Pill /Zhong Guo Bao Ji Wan.*

Another essential for the travel kit, this is an excellent remedy for digestive problems associated with food poisoning, with symptoms such as diarrhoea with stomach cramps, vomiting and flu-like feelings.

SAFETY FIRST

Work out your body type and requirements before taking any herbs.

Stop taking the herbs if you have any reactions to them. If these persist, consult your physician.

Always consult a doctor if you have any serious illness. Do not self-prescribe.

Do not take herbs alongside conventional drugs.

Never exceed the stated dose for a herb. It is a good idea to start with a small dose and work up.

Do not combine herbs in any way other than those suggested in this book.

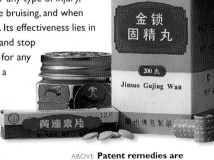

ABOVE **Patent remedies are a handy standby.**

99

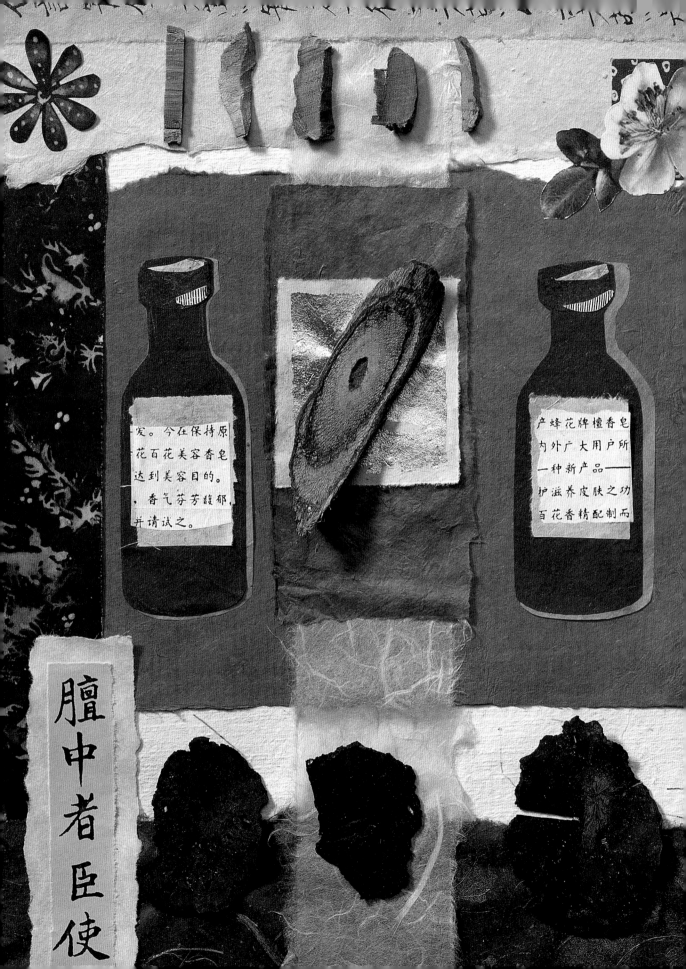

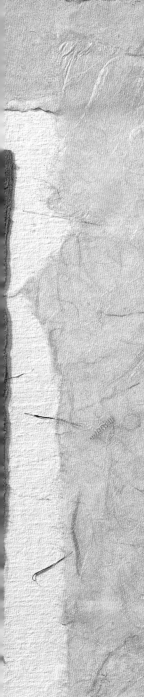

PART THREE

HERBS AND THEIR PROPERTIES

One of the basic reference works of any practising herbalist is a good *Materia Medica* (*Ben Cao* in Chinese). This is a book that lists all the herbs available and discusses their qualities, appearance and properties. There are some 5,000 different species of herb in China alone, and around 2,000 of these are used as medicines. Some are much more frequently prescribed than others, and a typical herbal dispensary will stock around 500 herbs. Here is a selection of commonly used herbs, known to be safe when taken as directed for the appropriate condition. There is also a section on herbs that grow in the West, for people who prefer to use indigenous plants.

WHEN IS A FOOD A MEDICINE?

The laws governing the sale of medicine and food are different. The legal situation will vary from country to country but often natural medicines are sold under food law. This means that they are not required to be licensed as a medicine, and there can be no hint of side-effects, as there is no concept in food law of what is referred to as a risk–benefit ratio. Herbs tend to be viewed by the authorities as unlicensed medicines.

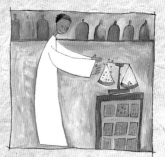

ABOVE **Herbs can be bought by mail order if they are hard to obtain locally.**

Treatment

However, only licensed medicines can make any form of claim about the product, including what it can be used for, or what it can treat. Unlicensed medicines are only labelled with the ingredients and any safety data.

Many of the herbs and spices used for medicinal purposes are also found in traditional cooking. So, when does ginger, for example, become a medicine? Adding chopped ginger to a stirfry is to use it as food. Slicing pieces of ginger into a tea with other herbs is a medicine. The same applies in Western herbal medicine – garlic is widely used as a food flavouring, but also as a medicine to combat heart and circulatory disease, colds and catarrh. The other main difference is that foods have a broad effect, while herbs have a much more specific action.

ESSENTIALS
There are many different methods of preparing dried herbs for a medicine.

Unlicensed medicines are not necessarily labelled with warnings about side-effects or contraindications.

ABOVE **Garlic crosses the boundaries: a ubiquitous food flavouring and a powerful medicine.**

HERBAL PREPARATIONS

Herbs are harvested, cured and dried. Depending on the type and part of the herb in question, the way in which it is prepared may vary.

DECOCTION

For a decoction, herbs are cooked with water for up to two hours. Decoctions are used for minerals, roots or thick bark, which require longer cooking times.
Advantages: the strongest way of taking herbs, the most 'field-tested' method, a minimal loss of the original herb qualities and potency.
Disadvantages: a laborious process, expensive as large amounts of herbs are required, strong-tasting and often unpleasant to Western palates.

INFUSION

To make an infusion, herbs are put into a teapot, boiling water is added, and the herbs are left to steep for several minutes. This method is only suitable for fresh or dried flowers and leaves, or herbs with a high volatile oil content. Infusions are widely used in Western herbal medicine, but are less popular in China.
Advantages: quick and easy to prepare, flowers and leaves usually taste pretty good.
Disadvantages: infusions have limited applications, and only certain herbs can be used.

DRAUGHT

For a draught, herbs are powdered, and cooked for 10–15 minutes; the liquid is then strained and drunk.

Advantages: most of the herbs that have to be decocted can also be prepared by this method. The cooking time is shorter than for a decoction, and smaller quantities of herbs can be used.

Disadvantages: requires a good-quality herb grinder, and each prescription must be ground to order.

TINCTURE

This method is particularly popular with European herbalists. A tincture is made by adding dried herbs to a quantity of alcohol and leaving it to steep for a period of time. The alcohol acts as a solvent for extracting properties from the herbs. This process is able to extract certain substances which could not be obtained by the water extraction method.

Advantages: easy to take and transport, good shelf-life, use of alcohol acts as a stimulant.

Disadvantages: strong-tasting, some aspects of the herbs lost in preparation, alcohol may be a problem for some people (although it can be evaporated off).

POWDERED HERB

POWDERED HERB IN CAPSULES

POWDERED HERB

TINCTURE (HERB IN ALCOHOL)

ABOVE **Tincture, powder and pills – various ways of taking herbs.**

POWDERED HERB FORMED INTO PILLS

RIGHT **To make an infusion, herbs are steeped in boiling water.**

CONCENTRATED POWDER

The process for making concentrated powders is relatively new, and similar to that used to manufacture instant coffee. The powder is taken mixed with water.

Advantages: easy to take and carry.

Disadvantages: strong and powdery taste, relatively expensive depending on the dosage, and some active constituents are lost in the production process.

PILLS AND CAPSULES

This is another traditional method of taking herbs, which has been updated by modern medical production technology.

Advantages: easy to take, no taste, transportable, good shelf-life.

Disadvantages: may be expensive depending on the type, large amounts have to be taken to achieve a high dosage, and it is impossible to alter the ingredients for each patient. The quality of ready-made pills and capsules is extremely variable, so it is important to always buy them from a reputable supplier of Chinese remedies.

Endangered species

In herbal medicine, the term 'herb' traditionally referred to any medicinal substance, whether plant, mineral or animal. Animals were utilized for curative properties, such as tiger bone for arthritis, musk deer for coma and rhino horn for fever. With the increasing popularity of oriental medicine, some animals have been driven close to extinction. Much of

the market is based on the mistaken idea that certain animal parts are aphrodisiacs. Many animals are now protected by the Convention on International Trade in Endangered Species, and it is illegal to sell them.

Check that your practitioner is registered with a professional body (see *page 184*).

CHINESE HERBS

In Traditional Chinese Medicine, plants, animal parts and minerals are used in remedies, although we refer to 'herbs' for convenience. All these healing substances are classified by their main therapeutic properties.

BAI ZHU

HERBS THAT STRENGTHEN THE QI

Ren Shen | Huang Qi | Bai Zhu
Dang Shen | Shan Yao | Ling Zhi
Da Zao | Zhi Gan Cao

HERBS THAT WARM THE BODY AND STRENGTHEN THE YANG

Du Zhong | Yi Zhi Ren | Gui Pi
Gui Zhi | Hui Xiang
Sheng Jiang | Hu Jiao | Hu Lu Ba
Ding Xiang | Wu Yao | Hu Tao Ren
Rou Dou Kou

HERBS THAT NOURISH THE BLOOD

Dang Gui | Shu Di Huang
He Shou Wu | Bai Shao Yao
Gou Qi Zi | Huo Ma Ren

HERBS THAT NOURISH THE YIN

Mai Men Dong | Yu Zhu
Xi Yang Shen | Bai He
Gou Qi Zi | Shu Di Huang

HERBS THAT AID THE DIGESTION

Chen Pi | Shan Zha
Mai Ya | Gu Ya | Shen Qu

HERBS THAT CLEAR DAMPNESS AND PHLEGM

Yi Yi Ren | Fu Ling | Sha Ren
Huo Xiang | Cang Zhu | Ze Xie
Chi Xiao Dou | Bei Mu | Xing Ren
Bai Jie Zi | Jie Geng | Kun Bu
Hai Zao

HERBS THAT ARE ASTRINGENT

Wu Wei Zi | Shan Zhu Yu
Wu Mei | Lian Zi | Fu Pen Zi

HERBS THAT CLEAR HEAT AND DETOXIFY

Jin Yin Hua | Lian Qiao
Ju Hua | Pu Gong Ying
Cang Er Zi | Huang Qin
Huang Lian | Huang Bai
Mu Dan Pi

HERBS THAT MOVE THE QI AND BLOOD

Chuan Xiong | Yu Jin
Yan Hu Suo | Tao Ren
Hong Hua | Dan Shen
Ji Xue Teng | Xiang Fu
Chai Hu | Qin Jiao | Du Huo

GOU QI ZI

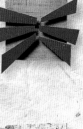

HERBS THAT CALM THE MIND AND SPIRIT

Suan Zao Ren | Yuan Zhi
Mei Gui Hua | Bai Zi Ren
Long Yan Rou

WESTERN HERBS

Aloe | Buchu Leaf
Chamomile | Cayenne
Chasteberry | Echinacea
Elderflower | Eyebright
Feverfew | Garlic | Ginkgo Biloba
Golden Seal | Hawthorn Fruit
Horsetail | Juniper | Marigold
Marshmallow | Milk Thistle
Nettle | Parsley | Passion Flower
Peppermint | Saw Palmetto
Slippery Elm | St. John's Wort
Valerian | Willow | Yarrow

Herbs that strengthen the Qi

Ren Shen I *Huang Qi* I *Bai Zhu* I *Dang Shen* I *Shan Yao* I *Ling Zhi* I *Da Zao* I *Zhi Gan Cao*

The Qi is the vital energy responsible for all the transformative and catalytic processes in the body. If there is insufficient Qi, the resulting symptoms will include tiredness, poor circulation, shortness of breath, poor digestion, low resistance to disease and reduced mental function. Herbs that are tonics for the Qi tend to be sweet-tasting and warming, which explains why we get sugar cravings when we are tired and run-down. Tonics should not be taken indiscriminately, or when not really necessary, or their boosting abilities will simply lead to Stagnation.

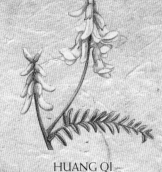

HUANG QI
Radix astragalus

This herb is becoming increasingly recognized for its ability to improve the action of the immune system. It is safe for many applications. Huang Qi is very sweet, and quite pleasant to take.

PROPERTIES
Sweet taste, slightly warm energy.

CHANNELS AFFECTED
Spleen and Lung.

ACTIONS
🌿 Strengthens the Lungs. For those prone to catching colds. For spontaneous sweating, tiredness and weakness.
🌿 Strengthens the Spleen. For diarrhoea, tiredness and weakness, weight loss, poor healing of the skin, oedema due to Deficiency of the Spleen.

DOSAGE
5–15g a day.

REN SHEN
Panax ginseng

This is a special, expensive herb that should be kept for occasions when its use is really warranted, such as when recovering from severe illness. Small amounts can also be used for a short period in winter to strengthen the Qi. It is one of the few herbs that is taken on its own as a revitalizer, either as a tea or in soup, and is also a frequent ingredient in formulas.

PROPERTIES
Sweet taste, slightly bitter, warm energy.

CHANNELS AFFECTED
Lung, Spleen and Heart.

ACTIONS
🌿 Replenishes the Qi. For fatigue and weakness.
🌿 Strengthens the Heart. For insomnia, palpitations and poor memory.
🌿 Strengthens the Spleen. For poor appetite, diarrhoea.
🌿 Strengthens the Lungs. For shortness of breath, dry cough.

DOSAGE
3–10g a day.

> **DO NOT USE** If there is high blood-pressure, for children under nineteen, during a cold, flu or virus.
> ——

> **DO NOT USE** Unless there are signs of Deficiency.
> ——

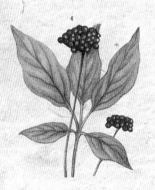

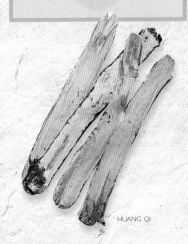

HUANG QI

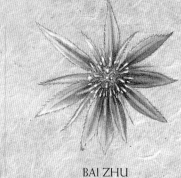

BAI ZHU

Atractylodes macrocephala

Bai Zhu is used for many problems affecting the digestive organs. It is well tolerated by the body, and has a moderate taste.

PROPERTIES
Sweet and bitter taste, warm energy.

CHANNELS AFFECTED
Spleen and Stomach.

ACTIONS
❀ Strengthens the Spleen and Stomach, tackling poor appetite, abdominal bloating, chronic diarrhoea. Aids resistance to disease.
❀ Clears Dampness and Phlegm – oedema and water retention due to Spleen Deficiency, Phlegm due to Spleen or Lung Deficiency.

DOSAGE
3–12g a day.

DO NOT USE When there is strong thirst due to Dryness or Heat.

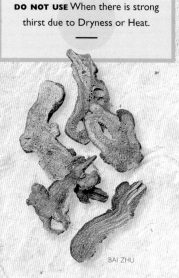

BAI ZHU

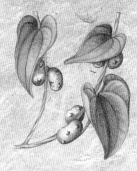

DANG SHEN

Codonopsis pilosula

Like most Qi tonics, this herb is fairly sweet and quite pleasant to take. It is very commonly used as a substitute for Ginseng, in cases where the strength of Ginseng is not required. Dang Shen is also a lot cheaper than Ginseng.

PROPERTIES
Sweet taste, warm to neutral energy.

CHANNELS AFFECTED
Spleen and Lung.

ACTIONS
❀ Strengthens the Spleen. For weakness of the limbs, poor appetite, loose bowels, Deficiency of the Blood.
❀ Strengthens the Lungs. For palpitations, shortness of breath and thirst.

DOSAGE
9–15g a day.

DO NOT USE During a cold, flu or virus.

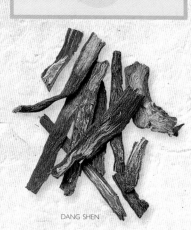

DANG SHEN

SHAN YAO

Dioscorea opposita

This is the root of the Chinese yam. Shan Yao works on both the Spleen and the Kidneys. Its effects on the Kidneys are responsible for its reputed hormonal actions. Shan Yao is neutral, and therefore well tolerated by the Spleen.

PROPERTIES
Sweet taste, neutral energy.

CHANNELS AFFECTED
Spleen, Lung and Kidney.

ACTIONS
❀ Strengthens Spleen, Stomach. For poor appetite, chronic diarrhoea, vaginal discharge.
❀ Strengthens Lungs, Kidneys. For dry cough, wheezing, frequent urination, bedwetting, impotence and infertility, seminal emissions.

DOSAGE
9–15g a day.

DO NOT USE When there is Full-Heat and toxins are present.

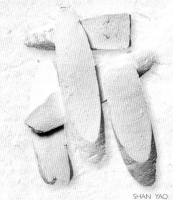

SHAN YAO

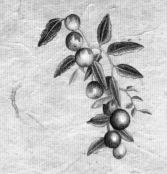
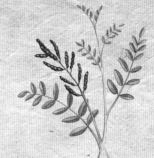

LING ZHI

Ganoderma lucidum

This is one of the famous 'mystical mushrooms' of Chinese Medicine. It is used today in a similar way to Huang Qi, as a stimulant for the immune system.

PROPERTIES
Sweet taste, slightly warm energy.

CHANNELS AFFECTED
Lung, Heart, Spleen, Liver and Kidney.

ACTIONS
🌿 Relaxes the Heart. For bouts of insomnia, palpitations, dizziness, poor memory.
🌿 Strengthens the Lungs. For shortness of breath, wheezing and a chronic cough.
🌿 Strengthens the Qi. For debility and weakness of the body.

DOSAGE
3–15g a day.

> **DO NOT USE** If there are no signs of Deficiency.
> ——

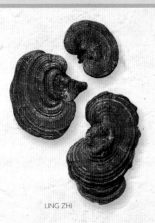

LING ZHI

DA ZAO

Ziziphus jujuba

This is the Chinese date, which can be eaten as a fruit or used in formulas. Dates are often added to any formula that is intended to act on the digestion, as they have a pleasant taste and are said to harmonize the formula.

PROPERTIES
Sweet taste and warm energy.

CHANNELS AFFECTED
Spleen and Stomach.

ACTIONS
🌿 Replenishes the Spleen and Stomach. For tiredness, poor appetite, Blood Deficiency, weight loss.

DOSAGE
3–6 fruits a day.

> **DO NOT USE** If there is a tendency to bloating or food intolerance.
> ——

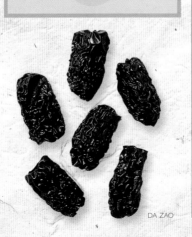

DA ZAO

ZHI GAN CAO

Glycyrrhiza glabra

Zhi Gan Cao is liquorice root, which has been specially prepared by baking it in honey. Liquorice is replenishing and detoxifying. This herb is often used to improve the taste of a formula, or to moderate its medicinal action.

PROPERTIES
Sweet taste and warm energy.

CHANNELS AFFECTED
Heart, Lung, Spleen and Stomach.

ACTIONS
🌿 Revitalizes the Heart. Treats palpitations.
🌿 Strengthens the Spleen. For weakness.
🌿 Strengthens the Lungs. For coughs and wheezing.
🌿 Protects the Stomach. Detoxifies poisons and moderates formulas. Soothes indigestion.

DOSAGE
2–9g a day.

> **DO NOT USE** When there is acute abdominal distension.
> ——

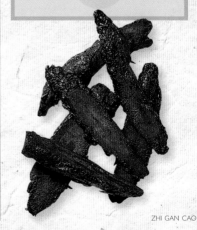

ZHI GAN CAO

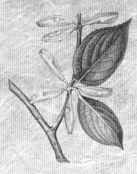

Herbs that warm the body and strengthen the Yang

Du Zhong I *Yi Zhi Ren* I *Gui Pi* I *Gui Zhi* I *Hui Xiang* I *Sheng Jiang* I *Hu Jiao* I *Hu Lu Ba* I
Ding Xiang I *Wu Yao* I *Hu Tao Ren* I *Rou Dou Kou.*

Yang energy is the basis of the Qi, so these herbs tend to be hotter and more deep-acting than the Qi-strengthening herbs. Many of them are also 'food-pharmacy' herbs, which are commonly found in the category of warming herbs, as they improve the flavour of food and aid digestion. If there is a tendency to Cold or Yang Deficiency, some of these can regularly be added to meals, particularly in the winter months.

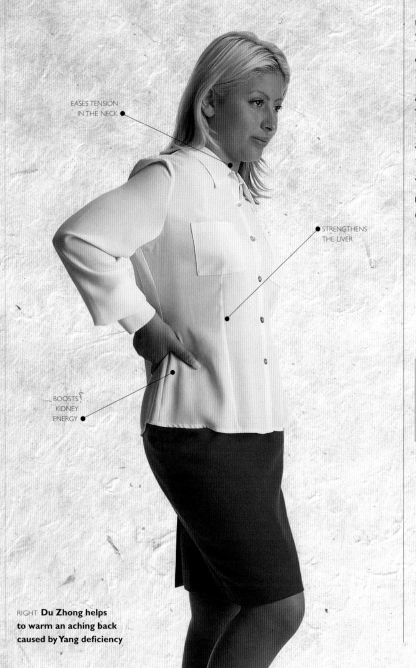

EASES TENSION
IN THE NECK

STRENGTHENS
THE LIVER.

BOOSTS
KIDNEY
ENERGY

RIGHT **Du Zhong helps
to warm an aching back
caused by Yang deficiency**

DU ZHONG

Eucommia ulmoides

Du Zhong is a bark. When it is peeled off the tree, it looks rather like snakeskin.

PROPERTIES
Sweet taste and warm energy.

CHANNELS AFFECTED
Liver and Kidney.

ACTIONS
❧ Strengthens the Liver and Kidneys. For lumbar aching and weakness, weak knees, frequent urination, impotence and threatened miscarriage.

DOSAGE
6–12g a day.

DO NOT USE If there is a pronounced Yin Deficiency.

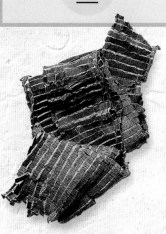

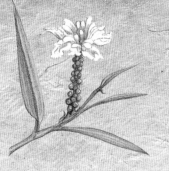

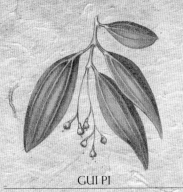

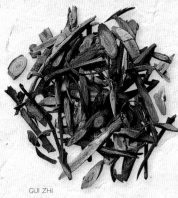

YI ZHI REN
Alpinia oxyphylla

This is one of the many types of cardamom used in Chinese Medicine, all of which have an action on the digestion and Water metabolism. Crack open the seed pod and gently stirfry the seeds before using them in a decoction. This will enhance Yi Zhi Ren's warming properties.

PROPERTIES
Pungent and warming.

CHANNELS AFFECTED
Spleen and Kidney.

ACTIONS
🌿 Warms the Kidneys. For frequent urination, urination at night and seminal emissions.
🌿 Warms the Spleen. For diarrhoea, nausea and poor appetite.

DOSAGE
3–9g a day.

DO NOT USE When there is vomiting or diarrhoea due to Heat.

GUI PI
Cinnamomum cassia

This is cinnamon bark. Rou Gui, Vietnamese cinnamon, is the most highly prized. However, Gui Pi is more than adequate for most conditions. It should be crushed or powdered and added only during the last five minutes of cooking time, or the oils will evaporate.

PROPERTIES
Pungent and warming.

CHANNELS AFFECTED
Heart, Liver, Spleen and Kidney.

ACTIONS
🌿 Warms the Spleen and Stomach. For digestive pain due to Cold, or poor digestion.
🌿 Warms the Kidneys. For lumbar pain and arthritis due to Cold.
🌿 Invigorates the Blood. For period pain.

DOSAGE
3–6g a day.

DO NOT USE When there is obvious Yin Deficiency or Heat.

GUI ZHI
Cinnamomum cassia

Gui Zhi (cinnamon twig) has some similarities to Gui Pui (the bark), but is used more to move the Qi and Blood and to open the pores of the skin. It is not as delicate as the bark, but do not cook it for more than fifteen minutes.

PROPERTIES
Pungent, sweet, warm energy.

CHANNELS AFFECTED
Heart, Lung and Bladder.

ACTIONS
🌿 Opens the pores to produce sweating. Good for chills, stiff neck and aching muscles.
🌿 Moves the Qi in the chest. For chest pain and palpitations.
🌿 Warms the circulation. For arthritis, joint pain due to Cold.
🌿 Promotes Blood circulation. For painful or obstructed periods.

DOSAGE
3–10g a day.

DO NOT USE When there is fever or Heat.

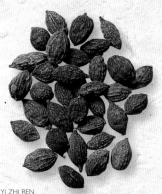

YI ZHI REN

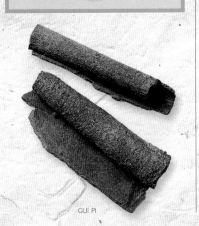

GUI PI

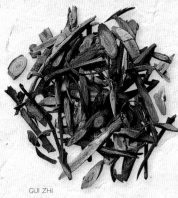

GUI ZHI

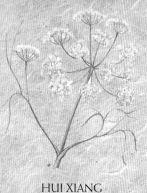

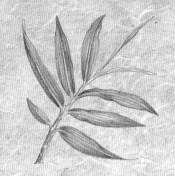

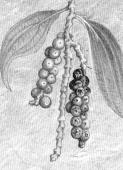

HUI XIANG

Foeniculum vulgare

This is a type of fennel seed, and like many herbs with combined medicinal and culinary uses, it can be used in cooking if it is appropriate to your body type.

PROPERTIES
Pungent and warming.

CHANNELS AFFECTED
Spleen, Stomach, Liver and Kidney.

ACTIONS
❧ Dispels Cold. For abdominal pain and distension due to Cold, including period pain, hernia pain and pain in the testicles.
❧ Warms the Spleen and Stomach. For poor digestion.

DOSAGE
3–8g a day.

SHENG JIANG

Zingiber officinale

This is fresh root ginger, one of the enduring tastes of the Orient. Dried ginger can be substituted at half the dose. It is an excellent remedy for nausea, taken as a tea.

PROPERTIES
Pungent and warming.

CHANNELS AFFECTED
Spleen, Stomach and Lung.

ACTIONS
❧ Warms the Spleen and Stomach. For nausea, vomiting and poor digestion.
❧ Opens the pores to produce a sweat. For a cold with cough and nasal discharge.
❧ Dispels Cold. For abdominal pain due to Cold.

DOSAGE
3–10g a day.

HU JIAO

Piper nigrum

Black pepper has always been prized for its flavour and pungency. A small amount of aromatic spice, such as black pepper, stokes the Digestive Fire and aids digestion. Black pepper is the immature fruit of the plant: it is processed to make white pepper. Choose peppercorns for medicinal use. Finely powdered pepper may be used instead, but at half the given dose.

PROPERTIES
Pungent and warming.

CHANNELS AFFECTED
Stomach, Spleen and Large Intestine.

ACTIONS
❧ Warms the Spleen and Stomach and dispels Cold. For nausea, vomiting, diarrhoea and abdominal pain due to Cold.

DOSAGE
1–4g a day.

DO NOT USE When there is Yin Deficiency or Heat.

—

DO NOT USE When there is Yin Deficiency or Heat.

—

DO NOT USE When there is Yin Deficiency with Heat.

—

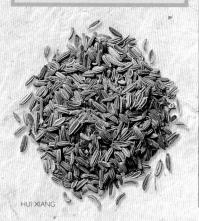

HUI XIANG

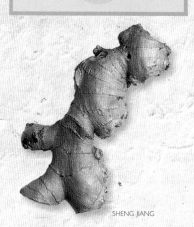

SHENG JIANG

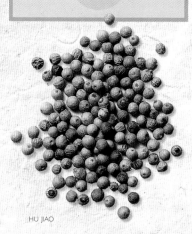

HU JIAO

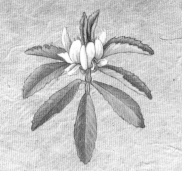
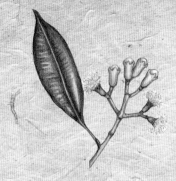
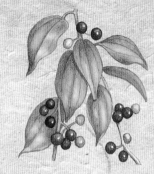

HU LU BA

Trigonella foenum-graecum

Hu Lu Ba, or fenugreek, is another of the warming food-pharmacy herbs, which improve the flavour of food and aid digestion. Fenugreek has been used in the East and Europe for thousands of years, both medicinally and in cooking. The Egyptians also used it for embalming. The seeds may be used medicinally.

PROPERTIES
Pungent with quite a bitter taste, warm energy.

CHANNELS AFFECTED
Kidney.

ACTIONS
⚘ Warms the Kidneys and dispels Cold. For abdominal or testicular pain that is worse with cold, hernia pain, lumbar soreness and oedema in the legs.

DOSAGE
3–9g a day.

DING XIANG

Eugenia caryophyllata

Ding Xiang, or cloves, are traditionally used in winter to help warm the body.

PROPERTIES
Pungent, warm energy.

CHANNELS AFFECTED
Spleen, Stomach and Kidney.

ACTIONS
⚘ Warms the Spleen and Stomach. For nausea, vomiting and hiccuping due to Cold.
⚘ Warms the Kidneys. For impotence and lumbar aches.

DOSAGE
1–3g a day.

WU YAO

Lindera aggregata

Wu Yao is a useful herb because it both moves the Qi and has warming qualities.

PROPERTIES
Pungent taste, warm energy.

CHANNELS AFFECTED
Spleen, Stomach, Kidney and Bladder.

ACTIONS
⚘ Warms the Kidneys. For frequent urination or the need to urinate during the night.
⚘ Dispels Cold. For menstrual pain due to Cold.
⚘ Warms the Spleen. For abdominal pain and distension due to blockage and Cold digestion.

DOSAGE
3–12g a day.

DO NOT USE When there is Yin Deficiency with Heat.

DO NOT USE When there are Heat symptoms and Yin Deficiency.

DO NOT USE When there is Full-Heat.

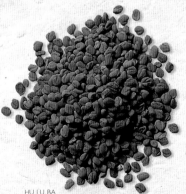

HU LU BA

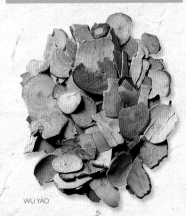

DING XIANG

WU YAO

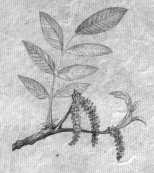

HU TAO REN

Juglans regia

Walnuts can be eaten on a regular basis by people who have a weakness of the Lungs or Kidneys, if they also have Cold symptoms.

PROPERTIES
Sweet taste, warm energy.

CHANNELS AFFECTED
Lung, Kidney and Large Intestine.

ACTIONS
🕉 Strengthens the Kidneys. For lumbar pain, weak knees, and frequent urination.
🕉 Stabilizes the Lungs. For cough and wheezing due to Cold.
🕉 Moistens the Intestines. For constipation due to Dryness.

DOSAGE
9–20g a day.

DO NOT USE When there are loose stools or Hot Phlegm.

———

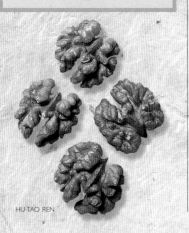

HU TAO REN

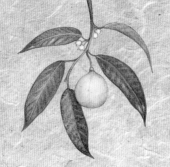

ROU DOU KOU

Semen myristica

Rou Dou Kou is good old-fashioned nutmeg. Like many other warming spices, it's a familiar taste from winter recipes. Nutmeg is native to Indonesia. The fruit of the plant (which also provides the spice mace) is used. Use only in medicinal amounts: nutmeg can be toxic – two whole kernels can kill.

PROPERTIES
Pungent taste, warm energy.

CHANNELS AFFECTED
Spleen, Stomach and Large Intestine.

ACTIONS
🕉 Warms the Spleen. For chronic loose stools, early-morning diarrhoea.
🕉 Warms the Stomach. For nausea and vomiting due to Stomach Cold and weakness.

DOSAGE
3–6g a day.

DO NOT USE For sudden diarrhoea due to food poisoning (or travel). Do not exceed the stated dose.

———

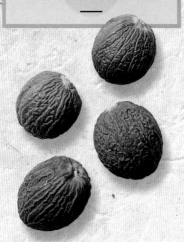

REMEDY

———

SI SHEN WAN

Bu Gu Zi (Psoralea corylifolia) 9g
Wu Zhu Yu (Evodia rutaecarpa) 6g
Rou Dou Kou 6g
Wu Wei Zi 6g
Sheng Jiang 1g
Da Zao 3 pieces

This traditional formula is used to warm the Kidneys and Spleen. Symptoms of weakness in the Kidneys and Spleen include early-morning diarrhoea, sometimes called 'cock crow' diarrhoea in China. Sufferers will also typically feel cold, tired and generally weak with a poor appetite, a pale tongue and a Deep, Slow pulse. Jujube dates (Da Zao) are often added to Chinese herbal prescriptions to modify and harmonize the mixture. As the method for making these pills is quite complex, it is recommended that you purchase them ready-made from a Chinese pharmacist.
• Dosage: follow the instructions on the packet.

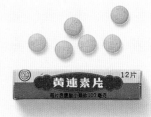

ABOVE **Patent remedies are ready-made classic formulas for curing common ailments.**

Herbs that nourish the Blood

Dang Gui I Shu Di Huang I He Shou Wu I Bai Shao Yao I Gou Qi Zi I Huo Ma Ren.

The Blood has many important properties, including the regeneration of tissue, the moistening of membranes and the cooling of the body. The emotions are also largely governed by the strength of the Blood, and several of the herbs in this category have soothing properties. They can be combined with herbs that calm the Mind to enhance this action. Herbs for the Blood are generally heavy and sticky and so can be slightly hard to digest. Therefore they should not be overused, particularly by people with a tendency to diarrhoea. The state of the Blood is said to be particularly important for women's health. When the Blood is in peak condition, it helps prevent problems associated with menstruation, pregnancy and the menopause.

HERBS FOR THE
BLOOD ARE
OFTEN COMBINED
WITH THOSE TO
CALM THE MIND

BELOW **To maintain
general good health
and keep the emotions
on an even keel, the
Blood needs to be
in peak condition.**

GOOD BLOOD
IS REFLECTED IN
A CLEAR SKIN

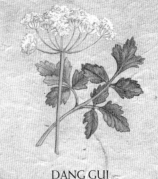

DANG GUI

Angelica sinensis

Angelica has very important medicinal qualities. It is sometimes referred to as 'women's Ginseng' because of its major role in the processes of the Blood, a substance of particular relevance to women.

PROPERTIES
Sweet and pungent
taste, warm energy.

CHANNELS AFFECTED
Liver, Heart and Spleen.

ACTIONS
❧ Nourishes the Blood. For all menstrual disorders and for Blood Deficiency.
❧ Invigorates the Blood. For pain due to trauma, chest pain and joint pain.
❧ Moistens the Blood. For constipation due to Dryness, dry skin, hair or nails.

DOSAGE
3–12g a day.

DO NOT USE If there is diarrhoea.
—

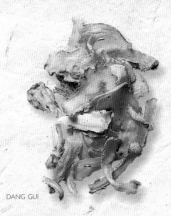

DANG GUI

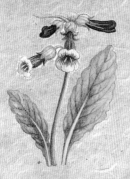
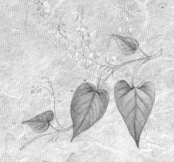
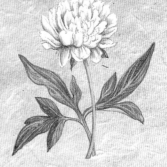

SHU DI HUANG

Rehmannia glutinosa

This is the prepared version of the Chinese foxglove, which will have been cooked nine times, for nine hours, before you buy it. It ends up looking like a slab of black leather and when used in a formula will turn the water black.

PROPERTIES
Sweet taste, slightly warm energy.

CHANNELS AFFECTED
Heart, Liver and Kidney.

ACTIONS
�</> Nourishes the Blood. For Blood Deficiency causing dizziness, palpitations, lack of periods.
🌿 Nourishes the Yin. For night sweats and hot flushes, dry skin, lumbar aching, infertility and impotence.

DOSAGE
9–20g a day.

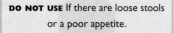

DO NOT USE If there are loose stools or a poor appetite.

HE SHOU WU

Polygonum multiflorum

The name of this herb translates as 'black-haired Mr Wu'. He Shou Wu is famed for improving the lustre and quality of hair. Greying hair can be a sign of Deficiency of the Blood, or it can indicate low Kidney energy.

PROPERTIES
Sweet and bitter taste, astringent action, slightly warm energy.

CHANNELS AFFECTED
Liver and Kidney.

ACTIONS
🌿 Replenishes the Liver and Kidneys. For greying hair, dry skin, weak knees and back.
🌿 Nourishes the Blood. For insomnia, palpitations and Blood Deficiency.
🌿 Moistens. For constipation due to Dryness.

DOSAGE
9–20g a day.

DO NOT USE When there is severe diarrhoea.

BAI SHAO YAO

Paeonia lactiflora

Bai Shao Yao is another major tonic herb for the Blood, and it is frequently combined with Dang Gui to complement its sour, cooling properties.

PROPERTIES
Sour and bitter taste, cool energy.

CHANNELS AFFECTED
Liver and Spleen.

ACTIONS
🌿 Calms the Liver. For headache due to Liver Excess, dizziness, irritability, mood swings.
🌿 Nourishes the Blood. For menstrual problems, heavy bleeding.
🌿 Relaxes the muscles and tendons. For cramps and spasms.

DOSAGE
9–18g a day.

DO NOT USE During acute abdominal pain due to Cold.

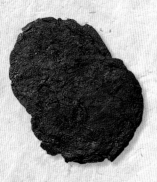

SHU DI HUANG

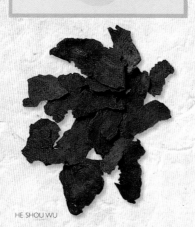

HE SHOU WU

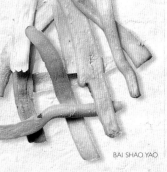

BAI SHAO YAO

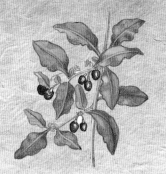

GOU QI ZI
Lycium barbarum

This small red fruit is also called wolfberry, because of its reputed ability to improve the vision.

PROPERTIES
Sweet taste, neutral energy.

CHANNELS AFFECTED
Liver and Kidney.

ACTIONS
🙶 Strengthens the Liver and Kidney. For impotence, weak back and knees.
🙶 Nourishes the Blood. For poor vision and dizziness.

DOSAGE
6–15g a day.

DO NOT USE When there is marked Spleen Dampness causing loose stools.

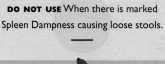

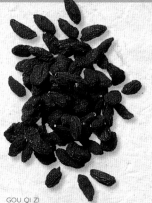

GOU QI ZI

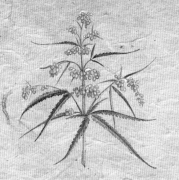

HUO MA REN
Cannabis sativa

Huo Ma Ren, or hemp seed, has been used for its medicinal properties for thousands of years. It is not psychoactive as it does not contain the chemical that produces the euphoria associated with the leaf. It is therefore legal in most countries. It is often combined with Bai Zi Ren. Hemp seed oil can be used externally on very dry skin, to help moisturize it. The seeds must be crushed before use.

PROPERTIES
Sweet taste and neutral energy.

CHANNELS AFFECTED
Spleen, Stomach and Large Intestine.

ACTIONS
🙶 Moistens the Intestines. For dry constipation, especially in the elderly.

DOSAGE
9–15g a day.

DO NOT USE If there is diarrhoea.

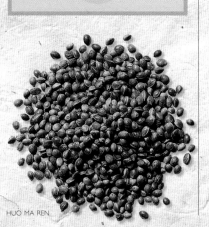

HUO MA REN

REMEDY
———

MA ZI REN WAN
HEMP SEED PILLS

Huo Ma Ren 20g
Bai Shao 10g
Xing Ren (Prunus armenica) 6g
Zhi Shi (Citrus aurantium) 6g
Da Huang 6g
Hou Po (Magnolia officinalis) 6g

These pills are available from Chinese pharmacists as a patent remedy for constipation in the elderly and weak, and also for those suffering from habitual constipation and piles. The mix is designed to clear Dry Heat in the Stomach and Intestines caused by a lack of fluids, so it has cooling and moistening properties. Sufferers will probably have a dry tongue with a yellow coating and a Floating, Rapid pulse.
• Do not take during pregnancy.
• Dosage: follow the instructions on the packet.

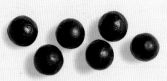

ABOVE **Pills for constipation are available from Chinese pharmacies.**

Herbs that nourish the Yin

Mai Men Dong I *Yu Zhu* I *Xi Yang Shen* I *Bai He* I *Gou Qi Zi* (see page 113)
Shu Di Huang (see page 112).

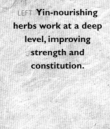

Yin is the source of Blood. These herbs have a deep action on the organs that produce the Blood. The cooling action of Yin herbs is stronger than that of Blood herbs, so they are used when Empty-Heat is generated because of Yin Deficiency. Like Blood herbs, Yin herbs are heavy and sticky, are slightly hard to digest, and should not be overused, particularly by people prone to diarrhoea.

LEFT **Yin-nourishing herbs work at a deep level, improving strength and constitution.**

LUNG CHANNEL

SOME YIN-NOURISHING HERBS, SUCH AS GOU QI ZI AND SHU DI HUANG, ALSO BOOST THE BLOOD

MAI MEN DONG
Ophiopogon japonicus

This herb works on the Blood and Body Fluids. Test it for quality by bending it between your fingers: it should not break when you bend it, and should feel moist.

PROPERTIES
Sweet and slightly bitter taste, with a cool energy.

CHANNELS AFFECTED
Heart, Lung and Stomach.

ACTIONS
❧ Enriches the Body Fluids. For a dry throat, thirst and for dry constipation.
❧ Moistens the Lungs. For dry coughs.
❧ Nourishes the Heart. For insomnia, palpitations and anxiety.

DOSAGE
6–12g a day.

DO NOT USE When there is Spleen Deficiency causing loose stools.

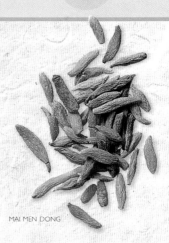

MAI MEN DONG

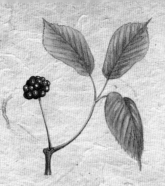

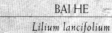

YU ZHU

Polygonatum odoratum

Yu Zhu is quite similar in action to Mai Men Dong, and can be used with it to augment Mai Men Dong's effects. It does not have any real effect on the Kidneys.

PROPERTIES
Sweet taste, cool energy.

CHANNELS AFFECTED
Lung and Stomach.

ACTIONS
☙ Enriches the fluids of the Lungs and Stomach. For dry cough, thirst, feelings of hunger.

DOSAGE
9–15g a day.

> **DO NOT USE** If there is distension of the epigastrium.
> ———

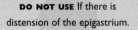
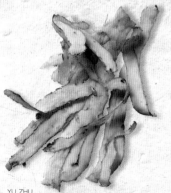

YU ZHU

XI YANG SHEN

Panax quinquefolius

Xi Yang Shen is American Ginseng, which has similar properties to Chinese Ginseng (Ren Shen), but is not warming. Therefore its action of promoting the Yin and Body Fluids is enhanced. However, it is even more expensive than Ren Shen.

PROPERTIES
Sweet and slightly bitter taste, cool energy.

CHANNELS AFFECTED
Heart, Lung and Kidney.

ACTIONS
☙ Nourishes the Yin and clears Heat. Effective for night sweats or afternoon flushes.
☙ Moistens the Lungs. For a chronic cough which is due to Lung Deficiency.
☙ Replenishing after illness.

DOSAGE
3–6g a day.

> **DO NOT USE** If there is poor digestion.
> ———

XI YANG SHEN

BAI HE

Lilium lancifolium

Bai He can be used with other herbs to treat the Lungs.

PROPERTIES
Sweet taste, cool energy.

CHANNELS AFFECTED
Heart and Lung. It also has a calming effect on the emotions.

ACTIONS
☙ Nourishes the Lungs. For coughs due to Empty-Heat, retained grief or sadness.
☙ Calms the Heart. Soothes the Mind and eases anxiety.

DOSAGE
9–15g a day.

> **DO NOT USE** For coughs due to Cold-Phlegm.
> ———

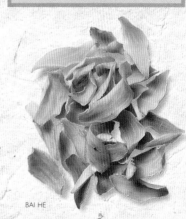

BAI HE

REMEDIES

YI WEI TANG

Sha Shen (Glennia littoralis) *6g*
Mai Men Dong *6g*
Sheng Di Huang *9g*
Yu Zhu (Polygonatum odoratum) *6g*
Bing Tang (rock sugar) *to taste*

This Stomach decoction (for the decoction method, see *page 100*) can be made up to replenish the Yin when Body Fluids have become depleted during fevers or influenza, or if there is Excess Liver Fire. Typical symptoms include a dry mouth, nausea, abdominal pains and dry, hard stools. The tongue is red, dry and has a thin coating; there will also be a Rapid pulse.
• Dosage: makes one dose. Take up to three times a day.

PING WEI SAN

Cang Zhu *6g*
Huo Po (Magnolia officinalis) *6g*
Chen Pi *3g*
Gan Cao *3g*
Sheng Jiang *1g*
Da Zao *3 pieces*

This neutralizing powder for the Stomach is used when there is Excess Damp in the Spleen and Stomach, with all the associated symptoms of bloating, loss of appetite, nausea, wind, acid regurgitation and diarrhoea. The mixture will dispel Dampness and will also regulate the circulation of Stomach Qi. The prescription is often modified by the addition of other herbs to deflect particular symptoms. Shen Qu and Mai Ya, for example, are added if there are symptoms of indigestion.
• Dosage: makes one dose. Take up to three times a day.

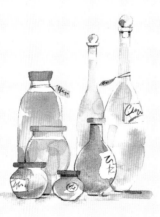

BELOW **Sipping an infusion of herbs can help with various problems. Pu Gong Yin is good for skin troubles, and Mei Gui Hua calms the Mind.**

● PU GONG YIN

MEI GUI HUA ●

Herbs that aid the digestion

Chen Pi I Shan Zha I Mai Ya I Gu Ya I Shen Qu.

A reduced digestive function, leading to food sensitivities or food intolerance, is very common. Food sensitivity seems to be a modern problem. Pollution and pesticides are two of the suspected culprits. These herbs address many of the symptoms such as bloating, tiredness after eating, nausea, gurgling innards, reduced appetite and loose bowel movements.

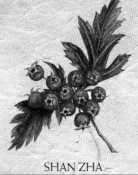

SHAN ZHA
Crataegus pinnatifida

Chinese Medicine primarily utilizes the digestive properties of Shan Zha, whereas Western herbal medicine tends to use it to increase blood circulation and reduce blood-pressure. Its action on blood-pressure is probably due to the herb's ability to reduce fat levels in the body.

PROPERTIES
Sour and sweet taste, slightly warm energy.

CHANNELS AFFECTED
Spleen, Stomach and Liver.

ACTIONS
🌿 Aids digestion. For bloating and indigestion from fatty food.
🌿 Regulates the Blood. Helps to reduce Phlegm and Dampness in the Blood.

DOSAGE
10–15g a day.

CHEN PI
Citrus reticulata

Chen Pi is a particular type of tangerine peel. Interestingly, although the flesh of oranges and tangerines is considered to produce Phlegm and irritate the digestion, the peel can be very beneficial. When used with other herbs that clear Phlegm, Chen Pi will augment their action.

PROPERTIES
Pungent and bitter taste with a warm energy.

CHANNELS AFFECTED
Lung and Spleen.

ACTIONS
🌿 Regulates the digestion. Used for bloating, distension, hiccuping, nausea and vomiting.
🌿 Clears Phlegm. For coughs with copious catarrh.

DOSAGE
3–9g a day.

PU GONG YIN INFUSION

MEI GUI HUA INFUSION

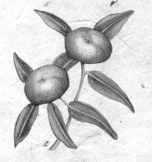

DO NOT USE For dry coughs or when there is bloody sputum.

DO NOT USE Unless there are symptoms of poor digestion and bloating.

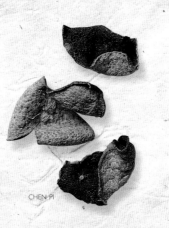

CHEN PI

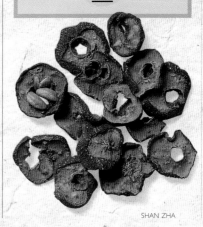

SHAN ZHA

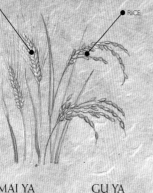

BARLEY • ● RICE

MAI YA   GU YA

Hordeum vulgare   Oryza sativa

These two herbs are, respectively, the germinated grains of barley and rice. It is interesting to note that these two plants help the digestion, because a lot of people with food intolerance are sensitive to grains. The difference is that by sprouting the plant, the energy changes to a more dynamic one. They can be used on their own (Mai Ya is stronger), but in practice they are often used together.

PROPERTIES
Sweet taste and neutral energy.

CHANNELS AFFECTED
Spleen and Stomach.

ACTIONS
🍂 Improves digestion. Helps to get rid of bloating, indigestion and poor appetite caused by eating grains and cereals.

DOSAGE
10–15g a day.

> **DO NOT USE** when breastfeeding – Mai Ya inhibits lactation.

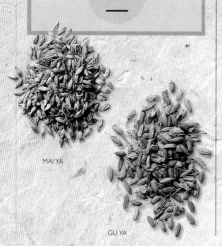

MAI YA

GU YA

SHEN QU

Massa fermantata medicinalis

This is actually a biscuit-like substance made from fermenting a mixture of six or seven herbs together. The exact formula varies according to the region of the country, or family tradition.

PROPERTIES
Bitter and pungent taste, with a warm energy.

CHANNELS AFFECTED
Spleen and Stomach.

ACTIONS
🍂 Harmonizes the digestion. Improves poor appetite. Helps to curb distension and bloating, gurgling innards and diarrhoea.

DOSAGE
5–15g a day.

> **DO NOT USE** During pregnancy or if there are symptoms of Heat in the Stomach.

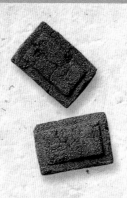

SHEN QU

REMEDY

____

LING GUI ZHU GAN TANG

Fu Ling 9g
Gui Zhi 6g
Bai Zhu 6g
Gan Cao 3g

This mixture of four major herbs is used as a warming decoction to clear Phlegm Stagnation. It will also strengthen the Spleen to resolve Dampness. Typically, it is used where Phlegm and Damp are due to a Deficiency of Spleen and Stomach Yang. This causes symptoms of vertigo, palpitations and breathlessness – conditions likely to be labelled chronic bronchitis or bronchial asthma by Western medicine. The tongue will have a white, slippery coating and the pulse is usually Slippery or Tight. If there is also nausea and vomiting, Chen Pi and Ban Xia are added to the mix to combat the rising Qi.
• Dosage: makes one dose. Take up to three times a day.

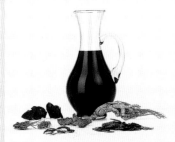

ABOVE **Decoctions are also known as 'tangs' – the Chinese word for soup.**

Herbs that clear Dampness and Phlegm

Yi Yi Ren | Fu Ling | Sha Ren | Huo Xiang | Cang Zhu | Ze Xie | Chi Xiao Dou | Bei Mu | Xing Ren | Bai Jie Zi | Jie Geng | Kun Bu | Hai Zao.

Dampness and Phlegm are considered to be a thickening of normal Body Fluids. Dampness affects the middle and lower parts of the body such as the digestive tract, Bladder and Kidneys, while Phlegm tends to be found mostly in the chest and head. However, anything that reduces Dampness in the middle of the body will tend to help clear Dampness or Phlegm above or below. This means that the digestive organs, particularly the Spleen, are often involved. Most of the herbs in this category have a relatively bland taste.

HERBS FOR DAMPNESS

Damp is described as turbid fluid. It is heavy and tends to sink downwards. Dampness impedes the normal functioning of the body as it tends to 'gum up the works'. It can also obstruct the normal flow of Qi, resulting in a lack of energy in the extremities or head. Dampness can easily be affected by, and tends to combine with, existing Heat or Cold in the body.

HERBS FOR PHLEGM

Phlegm can be seen as a stage further on from Dampness. It blocks rather than impedes, and can cause lumps in the organs or under the skin. It is harder to get rid of than Damp, and readily combines with Heat or Cold.

BELOW **Healthy meals, eaten sitting at a table, will help to combat Damp. Foods to avoid include dairy products and animal fats.**

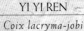

YI YI REN

Coix lacryma-jobi

Yi Yi Ren is Chinese barley, but pearl barley could be substituted if necessary, in a larger quantity. Barley can be added to foods if there is a tendency towards Dampness. Yi Yi Ren can be lightly stirfried before cooking (until just brown) to enhance its action on the digestion.

PROPERTIES
Sweet to bland, cool energy.

CHANNELS AFFECTED
Spleen, Stomach, Lung and Large Intestine.

ACTIONS
- Removes excess water from the body. Useful for difficult urination and oedema.
- Dries the Spleen. Effective for diarrhoea or loose bowels from Dampness in the Spleen.

DOSAGE
9–20g a day.

DO NOT USE During pregnancy.

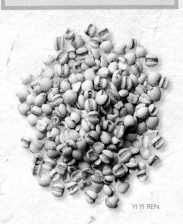

YI YI REN

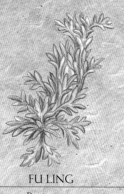
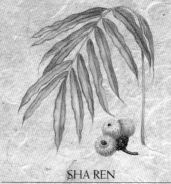
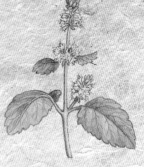

FU LING

Poria cocos

This rather odd herb is a type of fungus that grows around the roots of a particular tree.

PROPERTIES

Sweet or bland taste, with a neutral energy.

CHANNELS AFFECTED

Spleen, Lung and Bladder.

ACTIONS

Regulates water metabolism and removes Dampness. For oedema, difficult urination and abdominal distension.
Aids the Spleen. For diarrhoea due to Spleen Dampness.

DOSAGE

6–18g a day.

DO NOT USE When there is frequent urination.

SHA REN

Amomum villosum

Sha Ren is another type of cardamom. Its action relies on the volatile oils present in the seeds, so pods must be crushed before use and only added during the last ten minutes of cooking time. This herb is also said to 'calm the foetus', so it is a particularly good choice if there is morning sickness or a history of miscarriage.

PROPERTIES

Pungent taste, warm energy.

CHANNELS AFFECTED

Spleen, Stomach and Kidney.

ACTIONS

Resolves Dampness. For nausea, mild indigestion, abdominal distension, poor appetite.
Warms the Spleen and Stomach. For diarrhoea due to Spleen Deficiency and Cold.

DOSAGE

2–6g a day.

DO NOT USE When there is Heat in the Stomach.

HUO XIANG

Agastache seu pogostemon

Huo Xiang is the patchouli plant, highly prized in perfumery for its aromatic qualities. It is these pungent qualities that give the herb the ability to awaken the Spleen and resolve Dampness. Add during the last ten to fifteen minutes of cooking time, so the oils are not destroyed.

PROPERTIES

Pungent taste, slightly warm energy.

CHANNELS AFFECTED

Lung, Spleen and Stomach.

ACTIONS

For Dampness impeding the Spleen and Stomach, causing nausea, vomiting, morning sickness, bloating and distension, stuffy chest and reduced appetite.

DOSAGE

3–10g a day.

DO NOT USE If there is Heat in the Stomach.

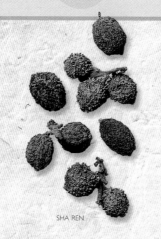

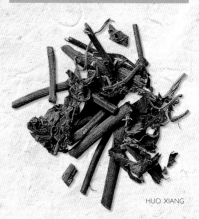

FU LING

SHA REN

HUO XIANG

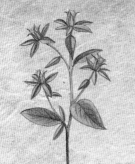

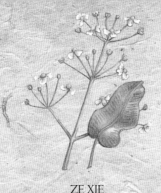

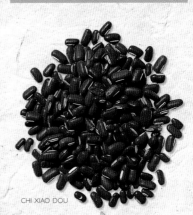

CANG ZHU
Atractylodes lancea

This is the same species as Bai Zhu (see *page 104*), Cang Zhu being 'grey' and Bai Zhu being 'white'. This herb is much more drying and does not have the strengthening action of Bai Zhu, but they can be used together if there is Dampness impeding the Spleen.

PROPERTIES
Pungent and bitter taste, with a slightly warm energy.

CHANNELS AFFECTED
Spleen and Stomach.

ACTIONS
Resolves Dampness in the Spleen. Useful for diarrhoea, nausea, abdominal distension, poor appetite and stiff joints due to Dampness.

DOSAGE
3–10g a day.

DO NOT USE Unless there are signs of Dampness.
———

ZE XIE
Alisma orientalis

Ze Xie is a type of water plantain. Its beneficial action is mostly on the urinary system.

PROPERTIES
Sweet or bland taste, cold energy.

CHANNELS AFFECTED
Bladder.

ACTIONS
Promotes urination. For difficult urination, retained urine, cloudy urine, oedema.
Clears Heat from the Bladder. Effective for burning urination, dark urine, bladder irritation.

DOSAGE
3–12g a day.

DO NOT USE If there is Cold or Yang Deficiency of the Kidneys, unless used with herbs to strengthen the Yang.
———

CHI XIAO DOU
Phaseolus calcaratus

Chi Xiao Dou, or Aduki bean, is a small red bean popular in many recipes. It is also often encountered as a sprouted bean. Here it is used for its diuretic action on Water metabolism. People with a propensity to Hot oedema can include it in meals.

PROPERTIES
Sweet and sour taste, with a neutral energy.

CHANNELS AFFECTED
Spleen, Heart and Small Intestine.

ACTIONS
Promotes urination. Useful for oedema, abdominal distension and urinary difficulty.
Clears Heat and detoxifies. Effective for swellings, jaundice and weeping skin lesions.

DOSAGE
9–20g a day.

DO NOT USE Unless there are symptoms of Dampness and Heat.
———

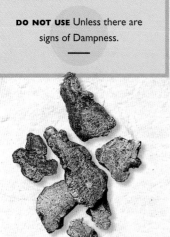

CANG ZHU

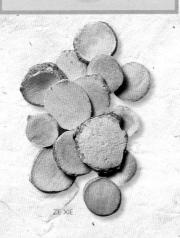

ZE XIE

CHI XIAO DOU

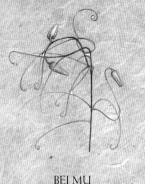
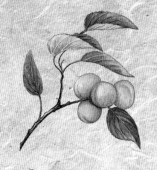
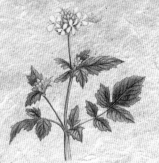

BEI MU
Fritillaria cirrhoza

There are two types of Bei Mu: Chuan (small), and Zhe (large). Their action is similar, but Chuan Bei Mu is more effective. This is a main herb for Hot-Phlegm in the Lungs, and for nodules and lumps.

PROPERTIES
Bitter and sweet taste, with a cold or cool energy.

CHANNELS AFFECTED
Lung and Heart.

ACTIONS
� Clears Hot-Phlegm from the Lungs. For a cough with sticky catarrh that is hard to expectorate and may be blood-streaked, chest tightness, or wheezing and cough with thick, yellow-green phlegm.
� Dissolves nodules. For swellings and abscesses in the Lungs, neck or breasts.

DOSAGE
3–9g a day.

XING REN
Prunus armenica

Xing Ren are apricot kernels. They taste similar to almonds, but are more bitter. They should not be eaten to excess.

PROPERTIES
Bitter taste, slightly warm energy.

CHANNELS AFFECTED
Lung and Large Intestine.

ACTIONS
� Stops coughing and wheezing. Best for a dry cough, but can also be combined with other herbs for a productive cough.
� Moistens the Intestines. For dry-type constipation.

DOSAGE
3–9g a day.

BAI JIE ZI
Sinapsis alba

Bai Jie Zi, or white mustard seed, is similar to horseradish. If you have ever eaten too much of this, you will be well aware of its ability to clear the nose!

PROPERTIES
Pungent, warm energy.

CHANNELS AFFECTED
Lung and Stomach.

ACTIONS
� Warms the Lungs to clear Phlegm. For a cough accompanied by copious white mucus.

DOSAGE
3–9g a day.

DO NOT USE For coughs due to Cold-Phlegm.

DO NOT USE In children or if there is diarrhoea. Do not exceed the maximum dose.

DO NOT USE When there is nausea or Heat.

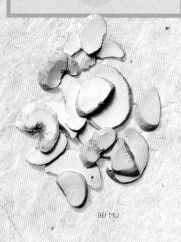

BEI MU

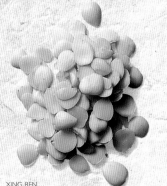

XING REN

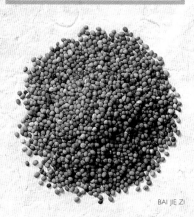

BAI JIE ZI

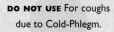

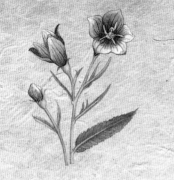

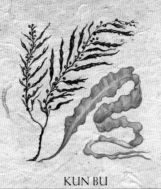

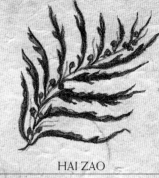

JIE GENG	KUN BU	HAI ZAO
Platycodon grandiflorum	*Laminaria japonica*	*Sargassum pallidum*

This is a major herb for relieving Phlegm in the upper body, and can be used for Hot or Cold Phlegm, depending on the other herbs it is combined with. Jie Geng also has a strong effect on the Lungs.

PROPERTIES
Pungent and bitter taste, with a neutral energy.

CHANNELS AFFECTED
Lung.

ACTIONS
🜊 Assists the Lungs. For a cough with yellow or white catarrh.
🜊 Benefits the throat. Relieves sudden soreness or inflammation of the throat.

DOSAGE
3–9g a day.

Kun Bu is kelp. In Western herbal tradition, kelp is used to increase the rate of the body's metabolism and has long been used as a treatment for an underactive thyroid. It is largely used, like sargassum, in the treatment of goitre, and for nodules in the neck associated with the presence of Phlegm.

PROPERTIES
Salty taste and cold energy.

CHANNELS AFFECTED
Spleen, Stomach and Kidney.

ACTIONS
• Reduces swellings – especially useful for oedema in the legs.
• Resolves and softens Phlegm nodules and lumps in the neck.

DOSAGE
3–9g a day.

There are two types of seaweed, kelp and sargassum. They are very similar in action and are often used together. Seaweeds have a particular affinity with the thyroid gland in the neck, due to their naturally high levels of iodine. Hai Zao can be bought as dried flakes. These can be powdered and used instead of salt – and will actually help to lower the blood-pressure.

PROPERTIES
Salty taste and cold energy.

CHANNELS AFFECTED
Spleen, Stomach and Kidney.

ACTIONS
🜊 Reduces Phlegm lumps. For swellings and obstructions in the neck or chest.
🜊 Benefits the Kidneys. Promotes urination, reduces oedema.

DOSAGE
9–15g a day.

DO NOT USE
No contraindications noted.

DO NOT USE If the Spleen and/or Stomach is Deficient or Cold.

DO NOT USE To excess if the Spleen or Stomach is Deficient or Cold.

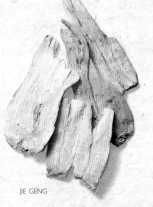

JIE GENG

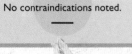

KUN BU

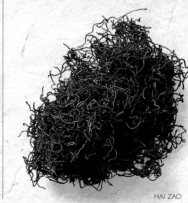

HAI ZAO

Herbs that are astringent

Wu Wei Zi | *Shan Zhu Yu* | *Wu Mei* | *Lian Zi* | *Fu Pen Zi.*

 The concept of astringency in Chinese Medicine is an interesting one. If a Body Fluid leaks out when it is not supposed to, it is because it has not been restrained by the appropriate organ. This can include diarrhoea or vaginal discharge (responsibility of the Spleen), urine or sperm (responsibility of the Kidneys and Bladder) and sweat (responsibility of the Heart or Lungs). Using one or more astringent herbs in a formula will help to restrain leakage. The predominant taste of astringent herbs is sour.

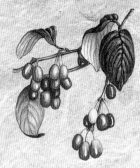

SHAN ZHU YU

Cornus officinalis

This small fruit has a specific action on the Liver and Kidneys.

PROPERTIES
Sour taste, warm energy.

CHANNELS AFFECTED
Liver and Kidney.

ACTIONS
🌿 Assists the Liver and Kidney Essence (Kidney Jing). For sore back and knees, dizziness, impotence, frequent urination, seminal emissions, spontaneous sweating.

DOSAGE
6–12g a day.

WU WEI ZI

Schisandra chinensis

The name of this fruit means 'five-flavoured seed', as it is considered to contain all Five Flavours (see *page* 37), although the predominant taste is sour. Because of this, Wu Wei Zi has some effect on all the Yin organs, and can also be regarded as a tonic herb.

PROPERTIES
Sour taste and warm energy.

CHANNELS AFFECTED
Lung, Heart, Kidney and Liver.

ACTIONS
🌿 Restrains the Lung Qi. For a chronic cough and wheezing.
🌿 Strengthens the Kidneys. For seminal emissions, incontinence of urine or faeces.
🌿 Controls sweating. For night sweats, spontaneous sweating.
🌿 Calms the Heart and Mind. For irritability, insomnia, palpitations.
🌿 Protects the Liver. Will help to relieve allergies.
🌿 Replenishes the body. Increases stamina and endurance.

DOSAGE
3–9g a day.

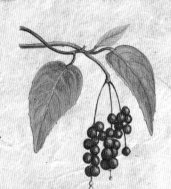

> **DO NOT USE** During a cold, flu or virus.

> **DO NOT USE** If there is urinary difficulty.

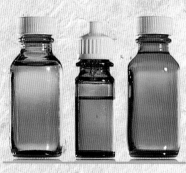

ABOVE **Astringents – shown here in tincture form – help to prevent the leakage of fluids.**

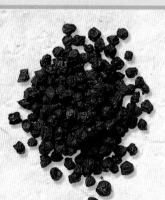

WU WEI ZI

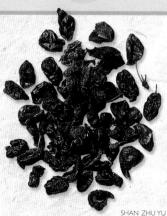

SHAN ZHU YU

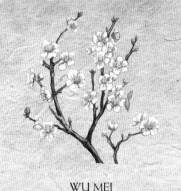

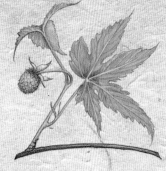

WU MEI

Prunus mume

This is a type of unripe black plum. As well as having an astringent action, this herb will kill certain intestinal parasites.

PROPERTIES
Sour taste, warm energy.

CHANNELS AFFECTED
Liver, Lung, Spleen and Large Intestine.

ACTIONS
🌿 Restrains the Lungs. Useful for a chronic cough.
🌿 Restrains the Spleen. Effective for chronic diarrhoea.
🌿 Consolidates the Body Fluids. Slakes the high thirst which results from Empty-Heat.
🌿 Kills intestinal parasites such as roundworm and hookworm.

DOSAGE
3–9g a day.

LIAN ZI

Nelumbo nucifera

Lian Zi comes from the lotus – a virtual pharmacy in itself, with five different parts producing medicinal substances. Lian Zi is the seed, or nut. To enhance its effect on the Spleen, lightly stirfry (until just brown) before decocting.

PROPERTIES
Sweet and astringent taste, with a neutral energy.

CHANNELS AFFECTED
Heart, Spleen and Kidney.

ACTIONS
🌿 Strengthens the Spleen. For chronic diarrhoea, poor appetite.
🌿 Consolidates the Kidneys. Helps to prevent seminal emissions and vaginal discharge.
🌿 Calms the Heart and Mind. Useful for insomnia, dream-disturbed sleep and palpitations.

DOSAGE
9–18g a day.

FU PEN ZI

Rubus chingii

Fu Pen Zi, raspberry fruit, is one of the joys of the berry season, with its distinctive sharp taste.

PROPERTIES
Sweet and sour taste, with a slightly warm energy.

CHANNELS AFFECTED
Liver and Kidney.

ACTIONS
🌿 Replenishes the Kidneys. Helps to prevent frequent urination, urination at night, seminal emissions, impotence, infertility.
🌿 Benefits the Liver. Useful for blurred vision.

DOSAGE
9–15g a day.

DO NOT USE During a cold, flu or virus.
—

DO NOT USE When there is constipation.
—

DO NOT USE When there is retention of urine.
—

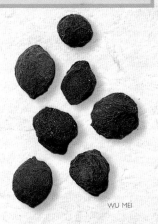

WU MEI

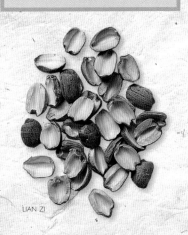

LIAN ZI

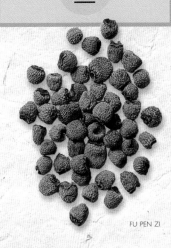

FU PEN ZI

Herbs that clear Heat and detoxify

Jin Yin Hua I *Lian Qiao* I *Ju Hua* I *Pu Gong Ying* I *Cang Er Zi* I *Huang Qin* I *Huang Lian* I *Huang Bai* I *Mu Dan Pi.*

This section combines several distinct areas in Chinese Medicine, covering herbs used to treat Heat, Damp-Heat, Blood-Heat and toxicity. They are listed under one section for ease of use, as their general actions are to cleanse and purify. Symptoms of toxicity in the body include skin disease involving discharges, pustules, purulent infections, itching, redness and heat. Many of these herbs have a bitter taste. The theory of the Five Elements and their associated Five Flavours tells us that the bitter taste belongs to Fire, and that the Heart is responsible for the complexion.

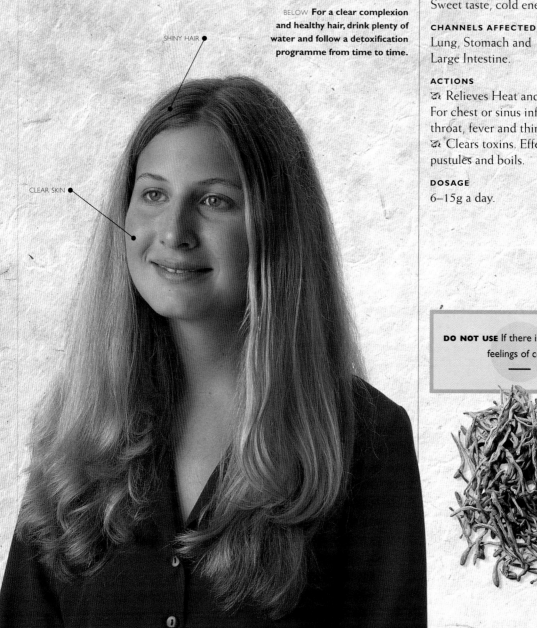

BELOW **For a clear complexion and healthy hair, drink plenty of water and follow a detoxification programme from time to time.**

SHINY HAIR

CLEAR SKIN

JIN YIN HUA
Lonicera japonica

Honeysuckle is known for its sweet nectar, and this is one of the few herbs in this section that does not have a pronounced bitter taste.

PROPERTIES
Sweet taste, cold energy.

CHANNELS AFFECTED
Lung, Stomach and Large Intestine.

ACTIONS
⚘ Relieves Heat and clears toxins. For chest or sinus infection, sore throat, fever and thirst.
⚘ Clears toxins. Effective for pustules and boils.

DOSAGE
6–15g a day.

DO NOT USE If there is weakness or feelings of cold.
—

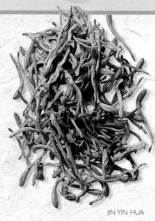

JIN YIN HUA

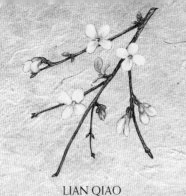
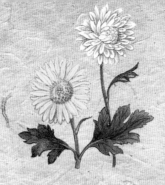
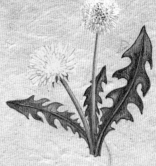

LIAN QIAO

Forsythia suspensa

Lian Qiao is the forsythia flower, which has a cleansing action. It is frequently combined with Jin Yin Hua for use in the early stages of a respiratory infection.

PROPERTIES
Bitter taste, cool energy.

CHANNELS AFFECTED
Lung, Heart and Gall Bladder.

ACTIONS
❧ Relieves Heat and toxins. For chest or sinus infection, sore throat, fever and thirst.
❧ Clears toxins. Useful for pustules and boils.

DOSAGE
6–15g a day.

JU HUA

Chrysanthemum morifolium

Ju Hua is chrysanthemum. There are several different types of chrysanthemum, but they are similar enough in action to be considered together. Ju Hua has a particular affinity with the eyes. It can be used on its own to make an infusion for relieving red or itching eyes. It is a pungent herb and should not be overcooked, or it will lose potency.

PROPERTIES
Pungent, sweet and bitter taste, with a cool energy.

CHANNELS AFFECTED
Lung and Liver.

ACTIONS
❧ Clears Heat. For a cold with fever, headache, red eyes.
❧ Calms the Liver. For temporal headaches, dry, red or itchy eyes.

DOSAGE
9–12g a day.

PU GONG YING

Taraxacum mongolicum

Pu Gong Ying is the dandelion-plant. It has been used for thousands of years in most herbal traditions. In Chinese Medicine, the parts growing above the ground are made into remedies, not the root. Pu Gong Ying has a particular affinity with the breasts.

PROPERTIES
Sweet and bitter taste, with a cold energy.

CHANNELS AFFECTED
Liver and Stomach.

ACTIONS
❧ Clears Heat and toxins. Effective for boils, weeping skin rashes and mastitis.
❧ Clears Damp-Heat from the Liver. For swollen and red eyes, and also for jaundice.

DOSAGE
10–20g a day.

DO NOT USE If there is diarrhoea, weakness, or feelings of cold.

DO NOT USE If there is severe diarrhoea.

DO NOT USE Unless there are symptoms of Heat and Dampness.

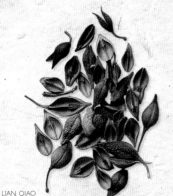

LIAN QIAO

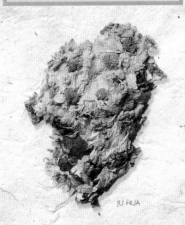

JU HUA

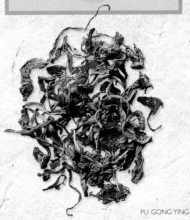

PU GONG YING

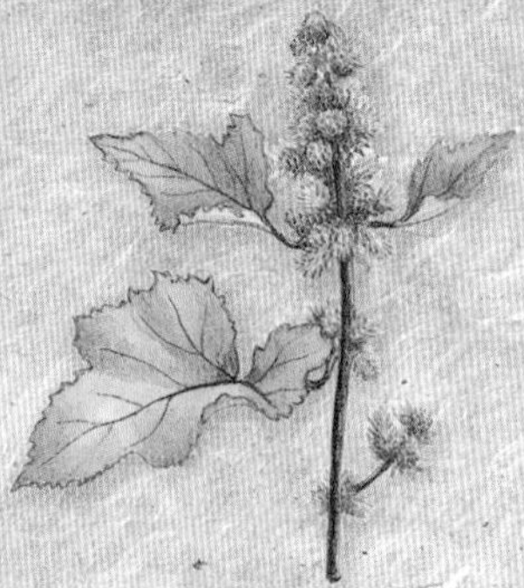

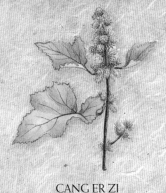

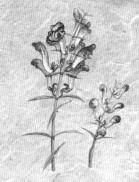

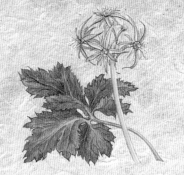

CANG ER ZI

Xanthium sibiricum

This herb has a particular affinity with the nose. Due to its particular properties, Cang Er Zi should always be cooked for at least 30 minutes before consumption.

PROPERTIES

Pungent and bitter taste, with a warm energy.

CHANNELS AFFECTED

Lung.

ACTIONS

- Opens the nose. For sinusitis and allergic rhinitis with thick discharge, plus associated headache.

DOSAGE

3–10g a day.

DO NOT USE For headaches due to Blood Deficiency.

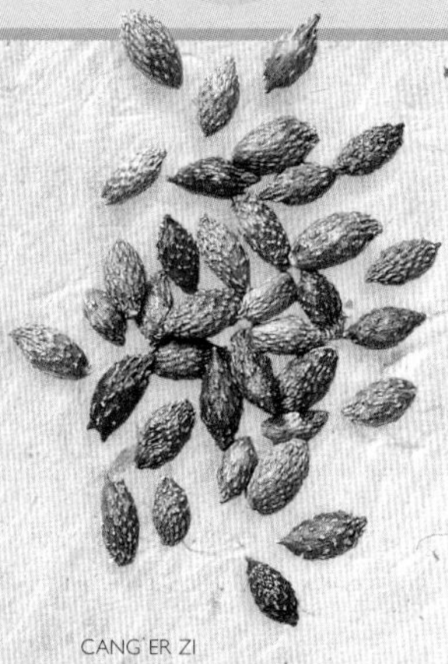

CANG ER ZI

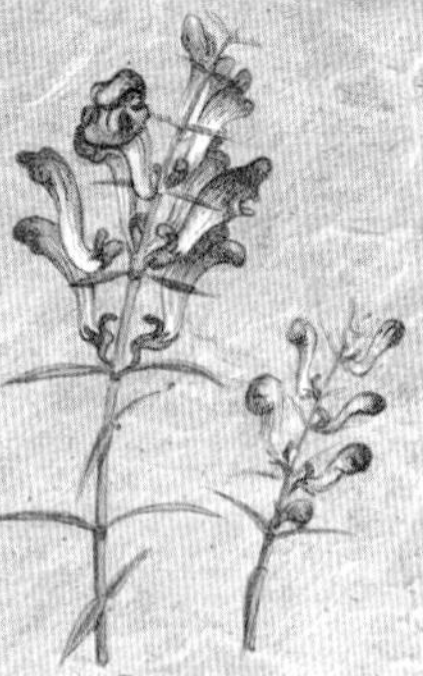

HUANG QIN

Scutellaria baicalensis

This is one of the herbs known as 'the three yellows' ('huang' means yellow). Huang Qin works on the upper body, chest, Lungs and Heart. It also 'calms a baby in the womb' when there is concern that it may be premature. When used for this purpose it should be lightly stirfried until brown.

PROPERTIES

Bitter taste, cold energy.

CHANNELS AFFECTED

Lung, Heart, Stomach and Gall Bladder.

ACTIONS

- Clears Heat and Dampness from the Lungs when there is thick yellow catarrh.
- For jaundice, urinary tract infections, diarrhoea from toxicity.
- Calms a baby in the womb.

DOSAGE

3–15g a day.

DO NOT USE If there are no symptoms of Heat and Dampness.

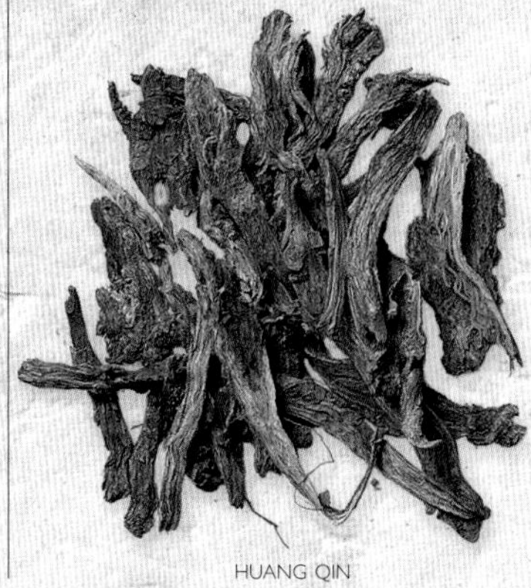

HUANG QIN

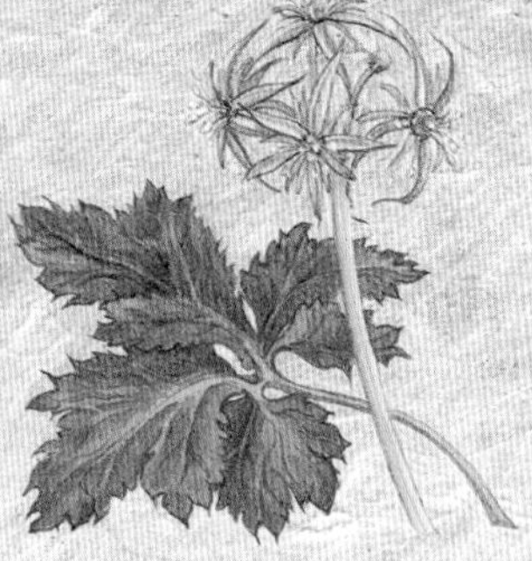

HUANG LIAN

Coptis chinensis

The second of the 'three yellows'. It acts mainly on the organs in the middle part of the body. It has been overused and is endangered. The European herb Hydrastis can be substituted for it.

PROPERTIES

Bitter taste, cold energy.

CHANNELS AFFECTED

Heart, Liver, Stomach and Large Intestine.

ACTIONS

- Clears Heat and Dampness from the Stomach and Intestines. For indigestion, acidity, reflux and diarrhoea due to Heat and Damp.
- Clears toxins. For red, inflamed eyes, ear and gum infections, inflamed and itching skin lesions.
- Clears Heat from the Heart. For insomnia and mania.

DOSAGE

1–6g a day.

DO NOT USE When there is diarrhoea due to Cold or Deficiency.

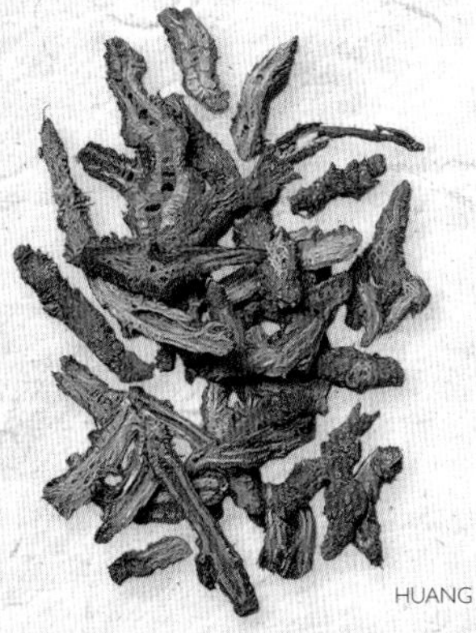

HUANG LIAN

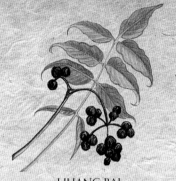

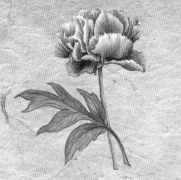

HUANG BAI
Phellodendron chinense

The third of the 'three yellows' exerts its main sphere of influence on the lower part of the body. Huang Bai also reduces Empty-Heat generated by Yin Deficiency.

PROPERTIES
Bitter taste, cold energy

CHANNELS AFFECTED
Kidney, Bladder and Large Intestine.

ACTIONS
🌿 Clears Heat and Dampness. For yellow vaginal discharge, urinary tract infections, diarrhoea due to Heat and Dampness.
🌿 Detoxifies. For wet skin diseases, boils and abscesses.
🌿 Clears Empty-Heat. For flushes and night sweats due to a Deficiency of Yin.

DOSAGE
3–10g a day.

> **DO NOT USE** For diarrhoea due to Cold or Deficiency.
> ———

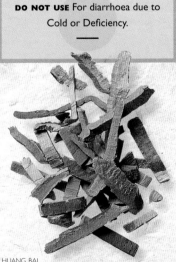

HUANG BAI

MU DAN PI
Paeonia suffruticosa

This herb cools the Blood. It also regulates the Blood when it has become Stagnant. During pregnancy, this should be used only in combination tonic formulas.

PROPERTIES
Pungent and bitter taste, cool energy.

CHANNELS AFFECTED
Heart, Liver and Kidney.

ACTIONS
🌿 Clears Heat from the Blood. For fever, nosebleeds or coughing of blood, bleeding under the skin, heavy and frequent menstruation.
🌿 Regulates the Blood. For painful periods, abdominal lumps due to Blood Stagnation.
🌿 Clears Liver Heat. For temporal headaches, red and painful eyes, flushed face.

DOSAGE
6–12g a day.

> **DO NOT USE** For Cold, or for sweating due to Yin Deficiency.
> ———

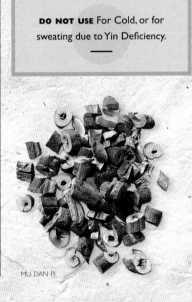

MU DAN PI

This is a classic Chinese prescription for replenishing Qi and strengthening the Spleen and Stomach. It is used where the Spleen and Stomach Qi are weak, leading to poor transportation of nutrients. Typical symptoms include a pale face, muscle weakness and digestive upsets with diarrhoea and vomiting – all symptoms of a weak digestion. Chen Pi may be added to the decoction to stimulate the flow of Qi.
• Do not use in Shi (Excess or Full) syndromes.
• Dosage: makes one dose. Take up to three times a day.

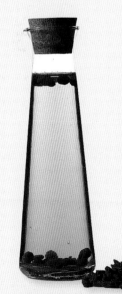

ABOVE **The traditional Chinese method for making decoctions and tinctures means that herbal properties are fully extracted.**

Herbs that move the Qi and the Blood

Chuan Xiong I *Yu Jin* I *Yan Hu Suo* I *Tao Ren* I *Hong Hua* I *Dan Shen* I *Ji Xue Teng* I *Xiang Fu* I *Chai Hu* I *Qin Jiao* I *Du Huo*.

When Qi and Blood are Stagnant, or do not flow smoothly and easily through the body, many symptoms can arise. In Chinese Medicine, all movement in the body is a manifestation of the flow of Qi, and pain is said to result from a blockage in the flow of Qi in the Meridians. Stagnation can also cause tightness, distension or emotional symptoms.

CHUAN XIONG
Ligusticum chuanxiong

This the root of a type of lovage. It has a particular action on both the head and the uterus.

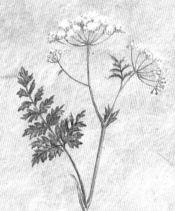

PROPERTIES
Pungent taste, warm energy.

CHANNELS AFFECTED
Liver, Heart and Gall Bladder.

ACTIONS
✿ Invigorates the Blood. For painful periods, abdominal masses due to Blood Stagnation, or chest or flank pain resulting from Blood Stagnation.
✿ Disperses Cold. For temporal headaches or joint pain due to Cold.

DOSAGE
3–9g a day.

> **DO NOT USE** In headaches due to rising Heat.
> ———

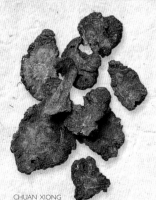

CHUAN XIONG

YU JIN
Curcuma wenyujin

Yu Jin is the spice turmeric, which is used extensively throughout the East, both in cooking and as a dye. It belongs to the same family as ginger. Powdered turmeric can also be dabbed on cuts and sores to speed healing time.

PROPERTIES
Pungent and bitter taste, with a cold energy.

CHANNELS AFFECTED
Lung, Heart, Liver and Gall Bladder.

ACTIONS
✿ Invigorates the Qi and Blood. For pain in the chest, flanks or abdomen, and period pain.
✿ Disperses Stagnation. For depression, mania, convulsions.
✿ Relaxes the Gall Bladder. For stones and jaundice.

DOSAGE
3–9g a day.

> **DO NOT USE** Unless there is Stagnation. Use with caution during pregnancy.
> ———

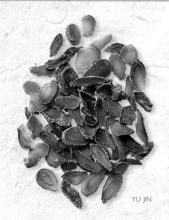

YU JIN

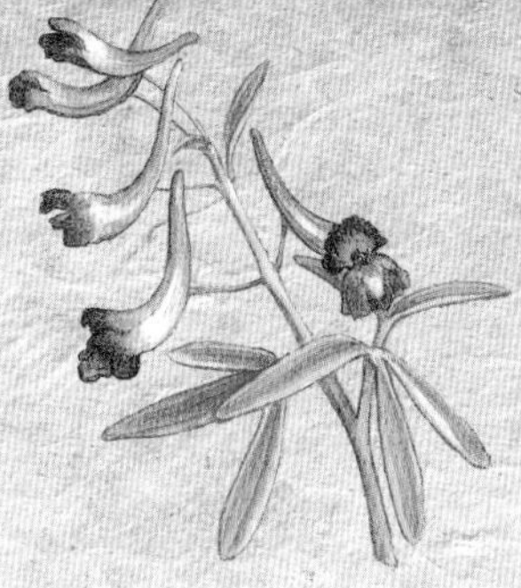

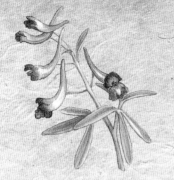

YAN HU SUO

Corydalis yanhusuo

Yan Hu Suo is generally regarded as the strongest analgesic (pain reliever) in the Chinese pharmacy.

PROPERTIES

Pungent and bitter taste, with a warm energy.

CHANNELS AFFECTED

Liver and Spleen.

ACTIONS

Moves the Qi and Blood. For pain due to trauma or Stagnation such as back pain, period pain, chest pain and abdominal pain.

DOSAGE

3–9g a day.

DO NOT USE During pregnancy, or for pain from causes other than Stagnation.

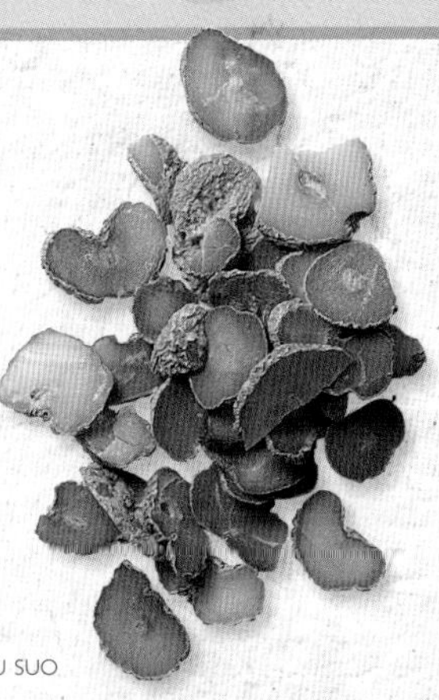

YAN HU SUO

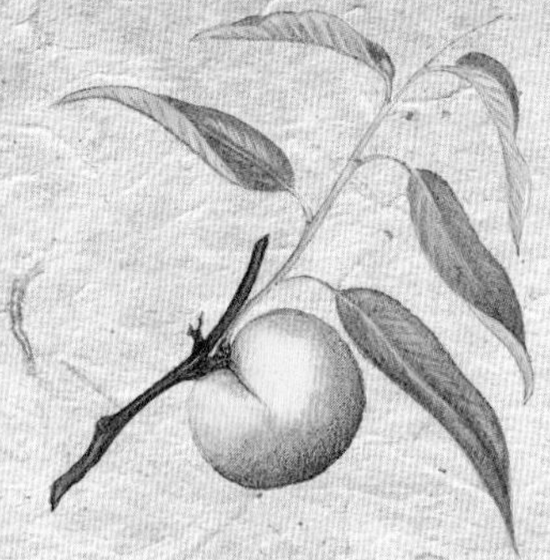

TAO REN

Prunus persica

Tao Ren, or peach seed, is used both to move the Blood and as a emollient for the Lungs and for the Large Intestine.

PROPERTIES

Sweet and bitter taste, with a neutral energy.

CHANNELS AFFECTED

Lung, Liver and Large Intestine.

ACTIONS

Moves the Blood. For pain due to Blood Stagnation.

Moistens the Lungs and the Intestines. For treatment of coughs and constipation.

DOSAGE

3–9g a day.

DO NOT USE During pregnancy.

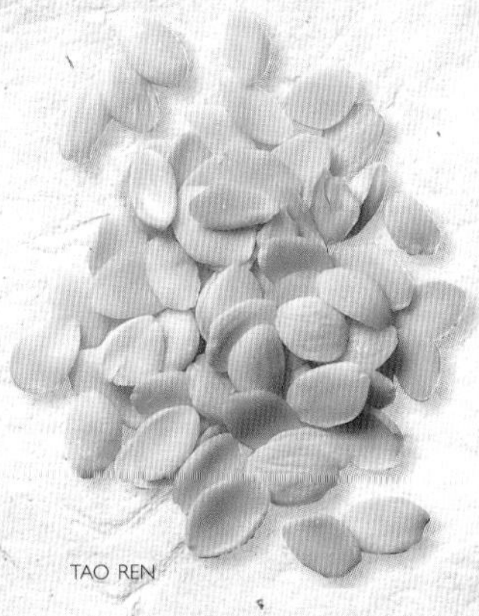

TAO REN

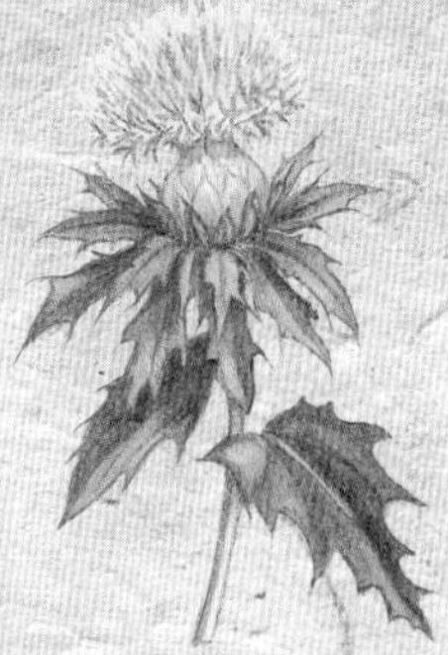

HONG HUA

Carthamus tinctorius

Hong Hua, or safflower, comes from the crocus plant. Crocus stamens are used to produce saffron, but safflower is a less expensive part of the plant. According to traditional Chinese Medicine theory, the action of substances accords with their appearance. Many of the herbs that work on the Blood have a vivid red colour, and it is this which partly explains their action.

PROPERTIES

Pungent taste, warm energy.

CHANNELS AFFECTED

Liver and Heart.

ACTIONS

Moves the Blood. Effective for pain caused by Blood Stasis, such as period pain, abdominal, flank or chest pain.

DOSAGE

3–9g a day.

DO NOT USE During pregnancy.

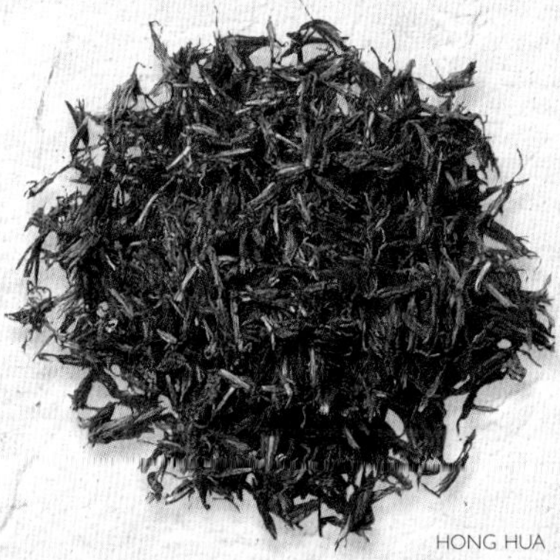

HONG HUA

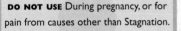

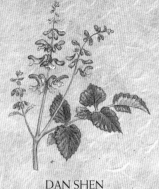
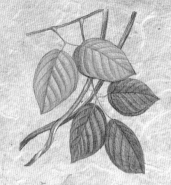

DAN SHEN

Salvia miltiorrhiza

Dan Shen is the red root of a type of sage plant.

PROPERTIES
Bitter taste, cool energy.

CHANNELS AFFECTED
Heart and Liver.

ACTIONS
🪶 Moves the Blood and clears Heat. Useful for pain or numbness due to Stasis, such as period pain and chest pain, pins and needles or numb extremities.
🪶 Regulates the Heart. Effective for insomnia and palpitations.

DOSAGE
3–15g a day.

JI XUE TENG

Spatholobus suberectus

Many of the Teng (or 'stem') herbs act on circulation to the extremities. Ji Xue Teng works on the legs, and on the Liver. The Liver regulates the flow of Blood, releasing more when the body needs it, such as during increased physical activity. When the demand for Blood subsides again, the surfeit is stored in the Liver. Thus it is important that the Liver functions efficiently.

PROPERTIES
Pungent and sweet taste, with a warm energy.

CHANNELS AFFECTED
Liver and Spleen.

ACTIONS
🪶 Nourishes the Blood and invigorates the circulation. For painful periods, joint pain and numbness of the limbs.

DOSAGE
6–15g a day.

XIANG FU

Cyperus rotundus

This is an important herb for regulating blocked Qi, both on a physical and an emotional level.

PROPERTIES
Pungent and slightly bitter taste, with a neutral energy.

CHANNELS AFFECTED
Stomach and Liver.

ACTIONS
🪶 Regulates the flow of Qi. For fullness in the chest or abdomen, flank pain, epigastric distension.
🪶 Regulates the menses. For period pain and PMS.

DOSAGE
6–12g a day.

DO NOT USE If there are no signs of Blood Stagnation.

DO NOT USE During pregnancy.

DO NOT USE When there are pronounced Heat symptoms due to Yin Deficiency.

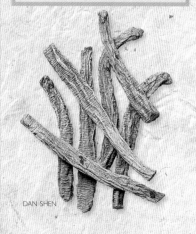

DAN SHEN

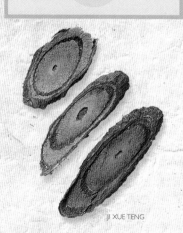

JI XUE TENG

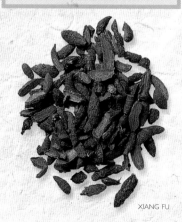

XIANG FU

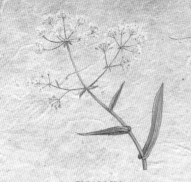

CHAI HU

Bupleurum chinense

Chai Hu is an interesting herb. It is generally classified as a Wind-Heat herb, which is a category of herbs used to treat colds and flu. However, Chai Hu also acts on the internal organs.

PROPERTIES
Bitter taste, cool energy.

CHANNELS AFFECTED
Liver and Gall Bladder.

ACTIONS
🕉 Regulates the Qi. For tightness in the chest, flank distension, mood swings, depression, PMS.
🕉 Alleviates fever. Effective when used for malarial-type alternating fever and chills.

DOSAGE
3–9g a day.

DO NOT USE Where there is Blood or Yin Deficiency, unless combined with tonic herbs.
——

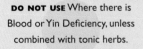

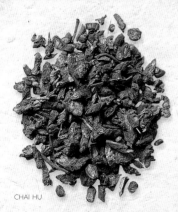

CHAI HU

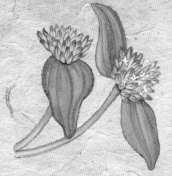

QIN JIAO

Gentiana macrophylla

Qin Jiao is used to treat Wind-Dampness – pain or stiffness due to changes in the weather. This herb is often combined with Du Huo. It mainly targets problems in the upper body.

PROPERTIES
Pungent and bitter taste, with a neutral energy.

CHANNELS AFFECTED
Stomach, Liver and Gall Bladder.

ACTIONS
🕉 Clears Dampness from the Channels. Useful for pain, aching, stiffness and cramping of the muscles and tendons.
🕉 Clears Empty-Heat. Use for 'afternoon fever' or low-grade chronic fever.
🕉 Moistens the Intestines. For dry-type constipation.

DOSAGE
4–12g a day.

DO NOT USE If there is chronic diarrhoea or frequent urination.
——

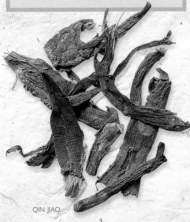

QIN JIAO

DU HUO

Angelica pubescens

Like Qin Jiao, Duo Huo is also prescribed for Wind-Dampness (pain or stiffness related to the weather). Both herbs are often combined. Duo Huo is more for problems in the lower body.

PROPERTIES
Pungent and bitter taste, with a slightly warm energy.

CHANNELS AFFECTED
Kidney and Bladder.

ACTIONS
🕉 Clears Dampness from the Channels. Useful for pain, aching, stiffness and cramping of the muscles and tendons.

DOSAGE
3–9g a day.

DO NOT USE When there is Heat or Yin Deficiency.

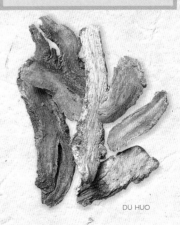

DU HUO

Herbs that calm the Mind and Spirit

Suan Zao Ren I *Yuan Zhi* I *Mei Gui Hua* I *Bai Zi Ren* I *Long Yan Rou.*

The most common translations for the concept of the Shen are Mind or Spirit, representing our mental and spiritual aspects and personality. The Shen resides in the Heart and encompasses the idea of intuitive thought, serenity and calmness. If the Heart does not house the Shen, mental and psychological disorders ensue. The ability to sleep soundly and the nature of dreams are particularly influenced by the Shen.

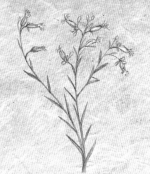

YUAN ZHI
Polygala tenuifolia

Yuan Zhi is another important herb for calming the Mind. According to Taoist thought, if the Mind is confused, Qi is weakened. Besides using herbs, techniques such as meditation help to calm and focus the Mind. The practice of Qi Gong, in which various postures are held, also helps to develop a meditative state, linking mental and physical aspects in keeping with holistic theory.

PROPERTIES
Pungent and bitter taste, with a warm energy.

CHANNELS AFFECTED
Lung, Heart and Kidney.

ACTIONS
❧ Calms the Mind. Useful for treating insomnia, palpitations, forgetfulness and anxiety.

DOSAGE
3–9g a day.

SUAN ZAO REN
Zizyphus jujuba

Suan Zao Ren is the small black seed of the wild date.

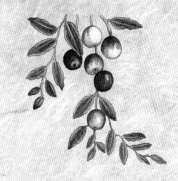

PROPERTIES
Sweet and sour taste, with a neutral energy.

CHANNELS AFFECTED
Liver and Heart.

ACTIONS
❧ Calms the Mind. For insomnia with dream-disturbed sleep or palpitations with anxiety.
❧ Restrains fluids. For night sweats or outbreaks of sweating.

DOSAGE
9–18g a day.

RIGHT **To achieve a healthy state of mind, give yourself time and space to relax, through methods such as meditation.**

> **DO NOT USE** If there is severe Heat present.

> **DO NOT USE** When there is Heat or Yin Deficiency.

SUAN ZAO REN

YUAN ZHI

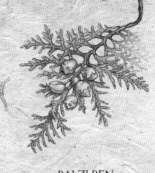

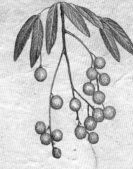

MEI GUI HUA
Rosa rugosa

Mei Gui Hua is the young flower of the Chinese rose. We tend to think of the rose as being the quintessential English flower, but in fact it was brought to England from China. Rose is much used in Western medicine in the field of aromatherapy, where the essential oil is particularly effective for treating menstrual problems, digestive troubles, depression, stress and insomnia.

PROPERTIES
Sweet and slightly bitter taste, with a warm energy.

CHANNELS AFFECTED
Liver and Spleen.

ACTIONS
☙ Regulates the Qi. Effective for tightness in the chest, period pain, depression and PMT.

DOSAGE
1–6g a day.

> **DO NOT USE**
> No contraindications noted.

BAI ZI REN
Platycladus orientalis

Bai Zi Ren is a similar seed to Huo Ma Ren (hemp seed), and is often combined with it.

PROPERTIES
Sweet taste and neutral energy.

CHANNELS AFFECTED
Heart, Liver, Kidney and Large Intestine.

ACTIONS
☙ Calms the Mind. For palpitations and insomnia with anxiety, due to Blood Deficiency.
☙ Moistens the Intestines. For dry-type constipation, particularly in the elderly.

DOSAGE
9–18g a day.

> **DO NOT USE** If there is diarrhoea or a lot of catarrh on the chest.

LONG YAN ROU
Dimocarpus longan

Long Yan Rou is a sweet, succulent Chinese fruit, not dissimilar to a raisin. People with Deficiency of the Blood, causing the symptoms listed below, can eat it as a fruit.

PROPERTIES
Sweet taste and warm energy.

CHANNELS AFFECTED
Heart and Spleen.

ACTIONS
☙ Strengthens the Blood and calms the Mind. Effective for insomnia, palpitations, forgetfulness and dizziness.

DOSAGE
6–12g a day.

> **DO NOT USE** If there is excess Phlegm or Dampness.

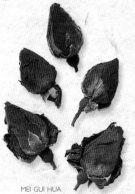

MEI GUI HUA

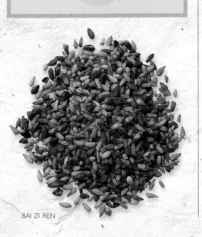

BAI ZI REN

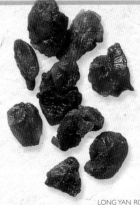

LONG YAN ROU

Western herbs

Aloe I *Buchu Leaf* I *Chamomile* I *Cayenne* I *Chasteberry* I *Echinacea* I *Elderflower* I *Eyebright* I *Feverfew* I *Garlic* I *Ginkgo* I *Golden Seal* I *Hawthorn* I *Horsetail* I *Juniper Berry* I *Marigold* I *Marshmallow* I *Milk Thistle* I *Nettle* I *Parsley* I *Passion Flower* I *Peppermint* I *Saw Palmetto* I *Slippery Elm* I *St. John's Wort* I *Valerian* I *Willow* I *Yarrow*.

The term 'Western herbs' is misleading. Many of the plants either originated in, or also grow in, the Orient. There are differences between the Eastern and Western attitudes to these herbs, and variations in soil and weather conditions have an effect on their properties. Modern Western herbal medicine analyses herbs to discover their chemical components, and this section will familiarize you with the main actions of these plants.

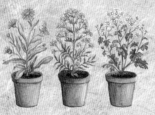

ABOVE **Herbs are easy to grow in pots; they are also attractive to look at and pleasantly scented.**

DOSAGE

These herbs are most freely available as tinctures or capsules, so the dosage recommendations on the bottle can be followed. Tinctures use alcohol as an ingredient, so if this is not desired (such as when treating children), drop the dose of tincture into freshly boiled water, leave for five minutes, and the alcohol will evaporate.

CONTRAINDICATIONS

Follow instructions on the packaging.

ALOE

ALOE
Aloe vera

Aloe is a type of cactus that grows in tropical countries. This plant has seen an astonishing rise in popularity in recent years, and many people take it on a daily basis as a tonic. This is a misconception. Aloe is not a tonic, but it does have detoxifying and cleansing properties. In Chinese Medicine, this herb is used as a laxative, and as with all such medicinals, habitual use will lead to dependency. It is inadvisable to take this or any other laxative on a regular basis.

The plant has two main parts: a clear green gel and a bitter yellow sap. The sap has the strongest purging qualities, so if you are buying bottled aloes, only use 'whole leaf' preparations for short periods.

USES
- For constipation.
- The elimination of parasites.
- Topical application for burns, rashes and itching.
- Detoxification of the stomach, large intestine and liver.

CONTRAINDICATIONS
- During pregnancy or if there is diarrhoea and weak digestion.

BUCHU LEAF
Barosma betulina

Buchu Leaf has a pleasant, black-currant flavour; it can be taken as a single herb infusion.

USES
- For acute cystitis with burning pain on urination.

BUCHU LEAF

CHAMOMILE
Matricaria chamomilla

Chamomile is an ancient anti-inflammatory remedy, which many people enjoy drinking as a tea. The slightly bitter taste is well worth acquiring.

USES
- For indigestion, ulcers, gastritis, flatulence.
- For an inflamed oral cavity or mucous membranes.
- For inflammation or itching of the skin.
- For an anti-spasmodic effect on abdominal cramps.
- For colic and teething in children.

CONTRAINDICATIONS
- Do exceed the stated dose (children especially).

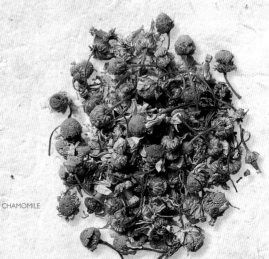

CHAMOMILE

CAYENNE

Capsicum minimum

Cayenne is red chilli powder, and so has warming and invigorating properties. Care must be taken to ensure the herb does not irritate the mouth or throat. This is particularly true if taken as a tincture, which is a very potent form of the herb.

CAYENNE

USES
- Strongly increases circulation to the extremities.
- Stimulates digestion.
- Stimulates the heart.
- Can be applied externally as a balm for joint pain.

CONTRAINDICATIONS
- Gastric acidity, gastric ulcers or highly elevated blood-pressure.

CHASTEBERRY

Vitex agnus-castus

The Chasteberry fruit is rumoured to have derived its name from its ability to lower the libido. However, another name for this herb is 'monk pepper', due to its apparent aphrodisiac qualities. This contradiction may be explained by the fact that the main action of Chasteberry is to balance the hormones, so either name can be applicable, depending on the existing disharmony.

USES
- Balances the hormones.
- Eases PMT/PMS and relieves symptoms of the menopause.
- Stimulates lactation.

CHASTEBERRY

ECHINACEA

Echinacea angustifolia

Originally a North American Indian remedy, this herb has a reputation for curative abilities. It is widely available as a tincture. It should not be taken continuously otherwise its effects will diminish. If used as a prophylactic, take only for two to four weeks at a time, leaving an equivalent gap before resuming. The plant is strongly anti-microbial and the root is often used in conventional Western medicine.

USES
- Stimulates the immune system to protect against infection.
- Anti-inflammatory in conditions such as tonsillitis and chest infections.
- Useful for countering poisons in boils, infections or abscesses.
- Reduces sensitivity to allergies.

ELDERFLOWER

Sambucus nigra

Both Elderflower and Elderberry are perennial remedies for colds and flu. They may be combined with Yarrow and Peppermint in an infusion. This remedy opens the pores, so after taking it, care should be taken not to get cold.

USES
- Promotes perspiration to clear colds and flu.

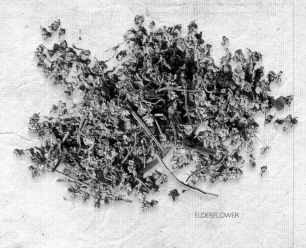

ELDERFLOWER

ESSENTIALS
If you grow your own herbs, make sure that you do not use pesticides.

After harvesting, herbs should be dried and stored in a container with a tight-fitting lid.

LEFT **Research has discovered that the leaves of *Echinacea purpurea* are just as effective as the root of *Echinacea angustifolia*. They can be used for the more convenient method of infusion, rather than having to make a decoction or tincture.**

ECHINACEA ROOT

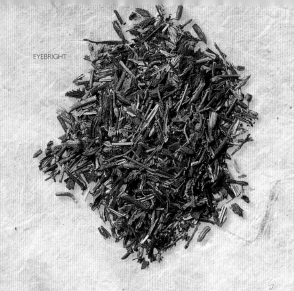
EYEBRIGHT

lungs appears to be due to the vaporization of the oils in the stomach, which then pass upwards. It is likely, therefore, that odourless Garlic capsules have a reduced capacity to fight infections.

USES

- Clears infection from the digestive and respiratory system in cases such as food poisoning, diarrhoea, chest infections and sore throats.
- Increases protection against infectious diseases.
- Kills parasites and fungal infections when used internally or topically.
- Increases the circulation and thins the blood.
- Detoxifies the gut.

EYEBRIGHT

Euphrasia officinalis

As the name implies, Eyebright is an important herb to 'brighten the eye'. It can be taken as a tea or the infused, strained liquid can be used as an eyewash.

USES

- Relieves inflammation and soothes the eyes.

FEVERFEW

Tanacetum parthenium

Feverfew has received a lot of publicity recently as a herb for migraines, and this reputation is largely deserved. Its action is due to the herb's vasodilatory effects (it opens the blood vessels), and it can therefore be used for inflammation of many sorts, as the name implies. It probably works best for burning headaches, where the pain is eased by the application of a cold pack.

USES

- Fights migraine and headache.
- Helps to relieve aches and pains resulting from inflammation.

FEVERFEW

GARLIC

Allium sativum

Garlic is the classic kitchen-pharmacy remedy, and it has been used all over the world for centuries as an antiseptic. Eating Garlic appears to lower blood cholesterol levels and protect the heart, and it also supplies vitamin C. The dosage can be increased to medicinal levels for an antibiotic effect (about 3–6 cloves daily for up to four days). Garlic's recognized action on the

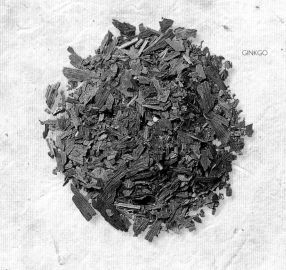
GINKGO

GINKGO

Ginkgo biloba

Ginkgo is another herb that has rocketed to fame recently, and is now the best-selling herbal remedy in the world. It has a strong vasodilatory action and the ability to increase circulation around the body. Also known as 'memory tree' for its ability to improve blood circulation to the brain, Gingko is now being used to treat degenerative memory disorders associated with age.

USES

- Effectively increases the peripheral circulation of the blood.
- Helps to counter reduced mental function, poor circulation and weak heart function.
- Stimulates and strengthens the flow of blood to the brain.
- Gingko seeds act on the Lung and Kidney Meridians and are often used in China for asthmatic disorders.

GARLIC

GOLDEN SEAL

Hydrastis canadensis

Golden Seal is one of the major 'bitter tonic' herbs. Bitter herbs stimulate the digestion and counteract sweet cravings, and have antiseptic and anti-inflammatory properties. Golden Seal stimulates the gall bladder to secrete bile, which assists in the process of digestion.

USES

🌿 Relieves infections and inflammations of the digestive tract, mouth, gums, gall bladder and liver.

🌿 Stimulates the digestion.

HAWTHORN

Crataegus laevigata

Both the flowering tops and the berries are used. The plant was originally used for kidney stones and as a diuretic, and later as a circulatory stimulant and heart remedy. It dilates the coronary arteries and increases blood flow, treating angina as well as mild congestive heart failure.

USES

🌿 Restores raised blood pressure to normal.

🌿 May be used with ginkgo as a boost for the cerebral circulation.

CAUTION

🌿 Consult your physician for all heart conditions.

HORSETAIL

Equisetum arvense

Horsetail has a diuretic effect on the kidneys. It also has blood-clotting abilities, which help in cases where the patient is spitting blood or has blood in the urine. The high level of silica in the plant appears to lend credence to its reputation for repairing connective tissue and healing wounds.

USES

🌿 For water retention, urinary infections and stones in the urinary tract.

🌿 Aids the repair of cartilage and connective tissue.

JUNIPER BERRY

Juniperus communis

This small pungent berry has a particularly strong diuretic effect on the kidneys.

USES

🌿 For water retention, oedema and retained urine.

🌿 For arthritic pain and swelling.

MARIGOLD

Calendula officinalis

Marigold is commonly available as an ointment for healing wounds and the skin, and stopping bleeding. This herb has antiseptic and anti-inflammatory properties. Internally, Marigold is used to combat inflammatory disorders of the digestive tract, including gastritis, peptic ulcers and colitis. It is also mildly oestrogenic and is a traditional remedy for a number of gynaecological complaints.

USES

🌿 Useful for unresolved infection, bleeding or erosion of the digestive tract, or enlarged lymph glands.

🌿 Use externally for fungal and other infections. It repairs the skin and can also be used as a mouthwash.

MARSHMALLOW

Althaea officinalis

Marshmallow is classified as a mucilage. This means that it is able to soothe the mucous membranes of the body. Roots, leaves or flowers are used. For indigestion, it is best taken as a powder cooked with hot milk, and can be mixed with other herbs, for example Slippery Elm and Liquorice.

USES

🌿 Effectively soothes the throat and lungs.

🌿 Helps to calm indigestion.

HAWTHORN

MARIGOLD

HORSETAIL

MARSHMALLOW

MILK THISTLE

Silybum marianum

Milk Thistle was originally used to stimulate lactation in nursing mothers. Recent research has indicated that one of its main constituents has a powerful effect on the liver, and this is now one of the herb's main applications.

MILK THISTLE

USES

🌿 Protects and detoxifies the liver and gall bladder, where there is accumulation of poisons or damage.

NETTLE

Urtica dioica

Stinging Nettles are rich in minerals and vitamins, and can be eaten in a salad or soup if scalded with boiling water to remove the sting. Do not eat plants that have grown by the side of the road, as they may be affected by traffic pollution. Nettles are highly nutritious and strengthen and cleanse the blood, as well as acting on the kidneys.

NETTLE

USES

🌿 Cleanses the blood in cases of toxicity or anaemia. Helps the kidneys remove uric acid from the body.

PARSLEY

Petroselinum crispum

Parsley counteracts wind. The plant, and particularly the seeds, have a strong stimulatory action on the uterus, helping it to contract. This should obviously be avoided during pregnancy, but can be useful when the birth is imminent and after giving birth. Parsley also has a strong effect on the kidneys. Like other plants which quickly rob the soil of its nourishment, Parsley concentrates many nutrients in its leaves and is a good source of vitamins and minerals.

USES

🌿 Stimulates the uterus.
🌿 Has a diuretic action in cases of oedema, gout, arthritis and kidney stones.
🌿 Parsley reduces acidity in the body.

PARSLEY

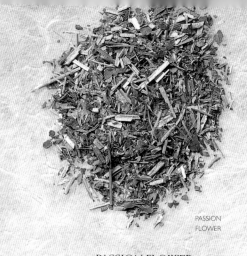

PASSION FLOWER

PASSION FLOWER

Passiflora incarnata

A major calming remedy. It can be combined with herbs such as Kava Kava – increasingly popular in the USA as a calming tonic – and Valerian. The aerial parts of the Passion Flower, which are strongly sedative, are used. The plant, of course, takes its name from the suggestion of Christ's Passion in its flowers, rather than for any more stimulating effect.

USES

🌿 For insomnia, anxiety, nervousness and depression.

PEPPERMINT

Mentha x piperita

Peppermint is best taken as a herb tea, as this preserves its volatile oils. This oil is extracted by steam distillation and is used in aromatherapy, mainly for colds and catarrhal conditions. The oil contains a high proportion of menthol, which can be extremely irritating to the mucous membranes, so Peppermint oil should not be used for babies and toddlers.

PEPPERMINT

USES

🌿 Useful for calming colic or gripe pain, flatulence, acidity, spastic colon, nausea and bilious attacks.
🌿 Has a generally relaxing effect on the mind.
🌿 Peppermint tea can help to relieve headaches and has a mildly anaesthetic effect on the skin. A few drops of the oil can be used in chest rubs for respiratory problems.

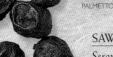

SAW PALMETTO

Seronoa repens

Saw Palmetto is now widely used for men's reproductive and prostate problems. This appears to have super-seded its traditional American Indian usage as a herb for catarrhal conditions. However, Saw Palmetto may also be used by women.

USES

❧ Supports the prostate and kidney in conditions such as benign prostatic hypertrophy, impotence, reduced sexual function and urinary infections.

SLIPPERY ELM

Ulmus fulva

SLIPPERY ELM

Slippery Elm is another excel-lent mucilage used to soothe the digestion. It can be combined with Marshmallow, as a powder, in hot milk.

USES

❧ Counteracts indigestion, acidity and reflux problems.
❧ For coughs and sore throats.

ST. JOHN'S WORT

Hypericum perforatum

St. John's Wort has a reputation as a restorative and relaxing herb. It has strong healing properties, but has attracted most attention recently for its action on mild to moderate depression, where it is thought to be as effective as anti-depressant drugs. Trials in Germany have demonstrated that it has far fewer side-effects than the popularly prescribed tri- and tetracyclic anti-depressants, and is also more effective than the fluoxetine group of drugs. The herb has also been used to stimulate the immune system in trials with AIDS patients.

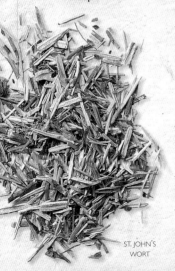

ST. JOHN'S WORT

USES

❧ Restores energy where tension and deple-tion are combined, such as when convalescing from long illness, or during the menopause.
❧ When used externally, it helps to promote the healing of tissue.
❧ Relaxes spasm and soothes tension.
❧ Relieves depression.

VALERIAN

Valeriana officinalis

Valerian is probably the strongest of the 'tranquil-lizer' herbs, as it acts on the central nervous system as a relaxant. It can be combined with Passion Flower for an enhanced effect.

USES

❧ Calms the nerves in cases of tension, spasm and nervousness.

VALERIAN

WILLOW

Salix alba

Aspirin was originally derived from the salicylic acid found in Willow. Its natural levels of salicin help to treat painful arthritic conditions. It is also possible that Willow exerts a similar blood-thinning action to aspirin, and so may be useful for heart conditions; consult your physician for advice.

USES

❧ For arthritis, joint pain.

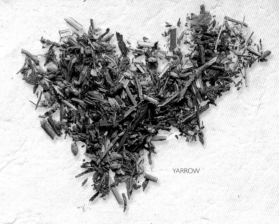

WILLOW

YARROW

Achillea millefolium

Yarrow is classed as a peripheral vasodilator, meaning that it boosts circulation to the extremities. This would seem to explain Yarrow's action in reducing moderate high blood-pressure, although care must always be taken with this condition.

YARROW

USES

❧ Dilates the blood vessels and increases circulation in cases such as varicose veins or hypertension.
❧ Helps to control fevers.

ALL THE TEA IN CHINA

Tea and China are indelibly linked. The infused leaves of the tea plant have been the main drink consumed by the Chinese for generations, both for refreshment and as a medicine. In Japan, the process of tea-making has been elevated to near mystical heights in the rituals of the tea ceremony. Tradition aside, modern research has confirmed that tea has a significant number of therapeutic properties and may increase resistance to certain types of cancer.

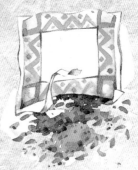

ABOVE **A cup of tea, taken without milk or sugar, will refresh your health.**

Tea types

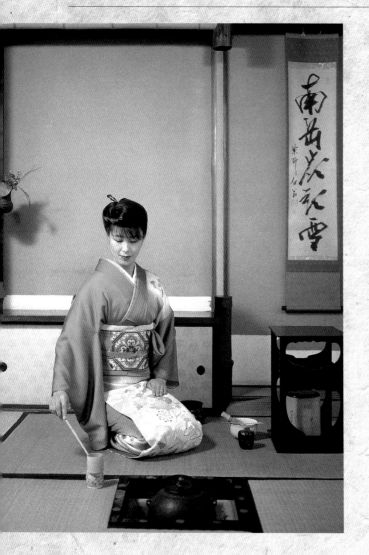

LEFT **In Japan, a ritualized ceremony has grown up around making and drinking tea.**

Tea makes up a substantial part of the European diet, and many Americans are now turning to tea as a healthier alternative to coffee, which contains a lot of caffeine. Tea also contains caffeine, but at much lower levels than coffee. People who are sensitive to caffeine are unlikely to have a problem with tea, especially if it is lightly infused.

Naturally, the Chinese have never added milk or sugar to hot tea, and if these two additions are left out, regular tea consumption can provide substantial health benefits. There are a great many kinds of tea available, and the common ones are outlined in the box. The two main types are black tea and green tea. In recent research, both have been shown to exert an antioxidant action on free radicals, the cells that can be responsible for cancer. This action is stronger in green tea, and only occurs when at least two or three cups a day are consumed. Black tea contains a higher level of tannins than green tea, and tannins have their own associated problems. According to some Chinese traditions, black tea is preferred for use in cold weather and is said to be warming, while green tea is cooler and therefore more suitable for hot days.

ESSENTIALS

There are various types of tea with different fermentation and drying processes.

———

Green tea is best drunk without milk or sugar. Two or three cups a day will have a significant effect on health.

GREEN TEA

The difference between green and black teas is fermentation. All tea is green until it is put through a curing or fermenting process, at which point most of the tannic acid and caffeine is produced. Green tea, like all teas, comes in many grades which can vary in price from almost nothing to hundreds of pounds a kilo. There is as much complexity and variety in the range of teas available as there is in fine wines. Experienced tea-tasters are rated as highly as 'nose' professionals in the wine trade. Luckily, even the cheaper grades of green tea are rich in properties that are beneficial to health.

DRINKING GREEN TEA

Green tea is the most suitable for daily drinking, and is best made with only a small amount of leaves, or even by pouring boiling water through tea held in a strainer. Mild green, jasmine or other black teas have a stimulating effect on the digestion if sipped while eating. Stronger preparations can be made by cooking tea for half an hour or more: this type of decoction can be used for conditions such as acute diarrhoea or chronic indigestion.

Drinking mild tea without milk or sugar is a taste that requires a little time to acquire, as some people find it slightly bitter to begin with. However, given its obvious health maintenance properties, it is clearly a habit worth acquiring.

Green tea

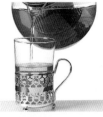

1 Put one teaspoonful of tea leaves into a teapot or tea strainer.

2 Pour boiling water into the teapot. If using a strainer, place it over a cup and pour the boiling water through.

3 Leave to infuse for a few minutes. Serve just as it is, without milk or sugar.

Types of Chinese tea

COLOUR/TYPE	EXAMPLES	FLAVOUR	CAFFEINE	BENEFITS
White	Sow Mee	very mild	none	refreshing
	Bojenmi	very mild	none	slimming
Green	jasmine	fragrant	slight	cooling
	gunpowder	bitter	slight	anti-carcinogenic, anti-cholesterol
	Loong Tseng	strongly bitter	slight	stimulating
	Lung Ching	delicate	slight	refreshing
	Tit Koon Yum	bitter	slight	stimulating
Oolong	Ti Kuan Yin	bitter	moderate	cooling, laxative
	Shui Hsien	bitter	moderate	cooling, laxative
Red	Puh-Erh	rich, pungent	moderate	digestive
Black	Ting Teh	rich, bitter	strong	stimulating
	Keemun	rich, bitter	strong	stimulating
	Boheas	rich, bitter	strong	stimulating

GINSENG ~ THE EMPEROR'S HERB

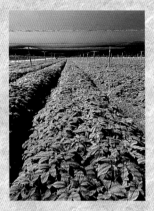

ABOVE **Commercially cultivated Ginseng, displaying the pink flowers of late summer.**

Ren Shen, or Ginseng, is probably the most famous tonic herb in the world. The quality of this herb is determined by its age and size, with the wild plants being most prized. Today, nearly all Ren Shen is cultivated — in fact it is the most expensive cash crop grown. The plant takes from three to seven years to mature. Genuine wild Ginseng, of an old age, would fetch a very good price indeed on the open market. Ginseng has been prized in Europe since the sixteenth century, and a root of it was famously given to Louis XIV (the 'Sun King') by a visiting delegation from the King of Siam.

Types of Ginseng

Various herbs are referred to as Ginseng, even those not of the Panax family (where Ren Shen, 'true' Ginseng, comes from). One thing most of these herbs have in common is that they have adaptogenic qualities. This means that they have the capacity to enable the body to adapt to many different types of stress. They all tend to be relatively expensive, with the exception of Siberian Ginseng.

REN SHEN
PANAX GINSENG | 'TRUE' GINSENG

This classic tonic herb is especially good as a tonic for the Qi. Ren Shen strengthens the function of the Spleen, Stomach, Heart and Lungs. It boosts the general constitution and raises immunity to disease. Although it is a stimulating and warming herb, it also promotes the production of Body Fluids. Ren Shen is one of the strongest plants in the herbal armoury, and it is precisely for this reason that it should not be consumed indiscriminately.

The appropriate uses for Ren Shen are the treatment of shock, during recuperation after a severe illness, and in small doses over a long period (by men over fifty) to sustain vitality. In younger people, particularly men, over-consumption of Ginseng can cause an over-excitation of the Qi leading to insomnia, anxiety, palpitations and restlessness.

The tannins found in tea and coffee are traditionally said to 'waste' Ginseng, and these drinks should be avoided while taking it. Because of these restrictions and its high price, Dang Shen is often substituted for Ren Shen, usually at twice the dose.

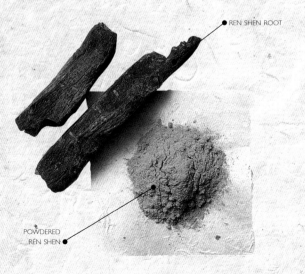

REN SHEN ROOT

POWDERED REN SHEN

CROSS CHECK *Ren Shen page 103, Dang Gui page 110, Xi Yang Shen page 115*

XI YANG SHEN ROOT

POWDERED XI YANG SHEN

POWDERED CI WU JIA

CI WU JIA ROOT

SAN QI ROOT

POWDERED SAN QI

DANG GUI ROOT

POWDERED DANG GUI

XI YANG SHEN

PANAX QUINQUEFOLIUS | AMERICAN GINSENG

This species originated in America. It is now cultivated in China, the biggest consumer of Xi Yang Shen in the world. It is harvested after three to nine years. Unlike Ren Shen, which is usually red in colour, American Ginseng is white and classified as a Yin tonic. It is therefore cooler and less stimulating than Ren Shen. Fluid-enhancing properties are particularly apparent in this variety. It is therefore especially useful for chronic dry coughs, as well as having the general qualities of Ren Shen. This herb is better suited to long-term consumption by younger people, and is a more appropriate choice for women.

CI WU JIA

ELEUTHEROCOCCUS SENTICOSUS | SIBERIAN GINSENG

Although not really a Ginseng or a true adaptogen, Siberian Ginseng appears to help the body to cope with difficult situations. It does not have the stimulating effects of real Ginseng, but can be used where there is Deficiency causing arthritis and joint pain. The plant was rediscovered in Siberia in the 1930s – hence the name – and it was once popular with Soviet athletes and lorry drivers as a means of improving stamina and resistance to stress. It is often used in the West to combat jet lag from long-distance travel.

SAN QI

RADIX NOTOGINGSENG | PSEUDO-GINSENG

San Qi is not really a Ginseng, but it is a valuable herb. This herb is unique in its effects on the Blood, having the ability both to stop bleeding and to regulate Blood flow. This action is useful in situations such as trauma due to injury or operation, where it is important to stop any further bleeding, while at the same time ensuring there is no blood clotting.

DANG GUI

ANGELICA SINENSIS | WOMEN'S GINSENG

This herb is sometimes referred to as a Ginseng as a sort of honorary title, due to its powerful effects on the Blood (a substance which, according to Chinese Medicine, dominates women's health). It is said to affect the Qi within the Blood, meaning that it is not only a Blood tonic, but also a Blood regulator. This is the mechanism behind Dang Gui's ability to correct many gynaecological conditions, which is emphasized in its name, meaning 'state of return', a return to normal periods.

ESSENTIALS

Many different plants are called Ginseng and each has quite different properties.

—

True Ginseng is an invigorating tonic. If used excessively, it can lead to over-excitation of the Qi.

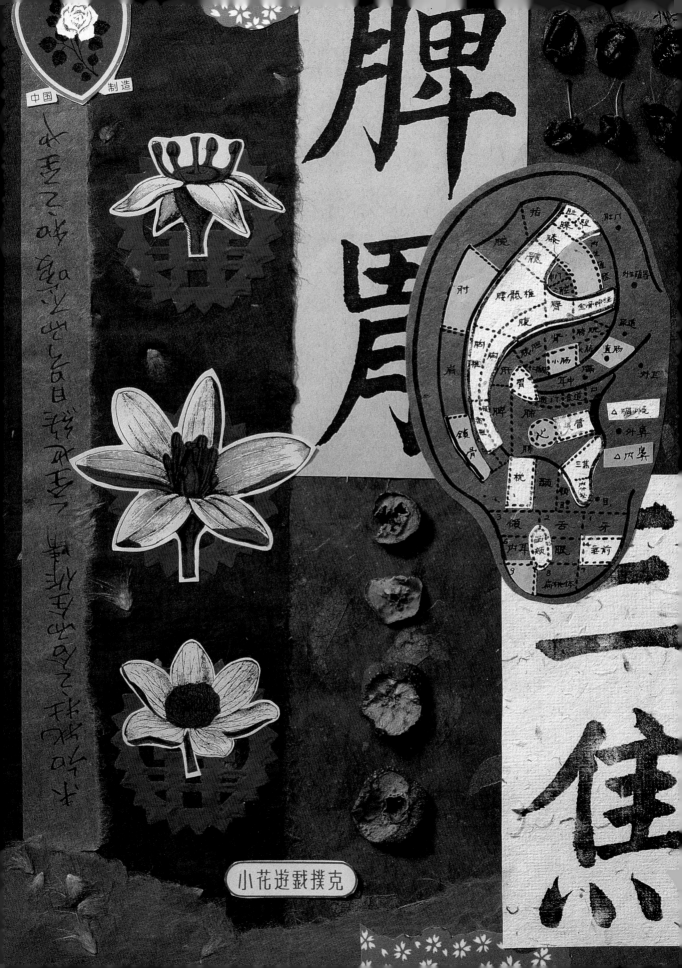

PART FOUR

USEFUL HERBAL FORMULAS

A complete understanding of Chinese herbal formulas is beyond the scope of this book. A doctor of Chinese Medicine will have studied for up to six years before prescribing herbs. But a lay person can learn how to combine small numbers of herbs as tonics or to remedy mild symptoms. In China there is a long tradition of the home use of herbs, and the average Chinese person has a reasonable working knowledge of the principles that lie behind Chinese Medicine. This section contains all the herbal formulas referred to in Part Two. There is also a selection of seasonal recipes and tonic wines to enjoy, and herbal creams and ointments to try out.

THE ART OF THE CHINESE HERBAL FORMULA

In China, systematic research and development over many generations has produced a medical tradition with a full theoretical and clinical background. The actions of the individual herbs are well understood, and this has led to a unique system of combining the herbs into special formulas. The use of formulas creates a synergistic energy, where the actions of the individual herbs are increased by combining them with others. The formula will be modified to suit the individual patient it is prescribed for.

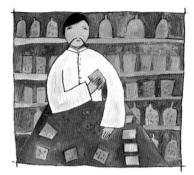

ABOVE **Chinese herbal suppliers keep a vast range of herbs in stock. These are weighed out to order. 'Herbs' also include minerals such as oyster shell or pumice.**

New tastes

Chinese Medicine has proved safe and effective when administered correctly, and is a powerful tool in the maintenance of health and the curing of disease.

Chinese herbs appear strange and exotic to us in the West, and at first we may find their taste and aroma unusual. However, it generally only takes a short time to adjust, and indeed people often find they actually crave the herbs! The process of cooking them may seem bothersome, but it is a step towards regaining control of our health. Allow yourself a week to get used to them, and you will find the process an enjoyable one. The various formulas are mixed into powders (San), pills (Wan), or decoctions (Tang), each with a highly descriptive name.

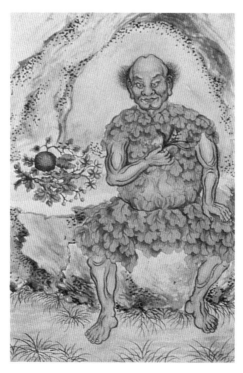

ABOVE **The mythical Shen Nong, the Divine Farmer, is credited with introducing the art of herbalism to the Chinese.**

SAFETY FIRST

Work out your body type and requirements before taking any herbs.

Stop taking the herbs if you have any reactions to them. If these persist, consult your physician.

Always consult a physician if you have a serious illness. Do not self-prescribe.

Do not take herbs alongside conventional drugs.

Never exceed the stated dose for a herb. It is a good idea to start with the smallest dose and work up.

Do not combine herbs in any way other than those suggested in this book.

MAKING A DECOCTION

Tang, meaning 'soup', is the word used to describe the traditional process of cooking dried herbs with water to make a decoction or tea. All Chinese households keep a special vessel for brewing medicinal soups.

DOSAGE

The decoction will provide between 2 and 6 doses.
- Low dose: divide the liquid into 6 doses.
- Medium dose: divide the liquid into 4 doses.
- High dose: divide the liquid into 2 doses.

If you have not taken the herbs before, start at the lowest dose, and increase it over a period of several days if the desired effect is not achieved with the lowest dose. Remember that herbs usually take some time to work – maybe months. For chronic conditions, try the herbs at a low to medium dosage, over several weeks.

- Drink one dose of the decoction, warm or at room temperature, twice daily.
- Drink the decoction about one hour or more after food, or about 30 minutes or more before food. If this is impossible, take it at your convenience.
- Do not drink the sediment. If you have not taken herbs before, have your first dose in the evening after food.

Making a decoction

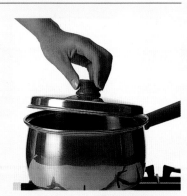

1 Put the herbs into a cooking pot (do not use aluminium or cast-iron). Add just enough cold water to cover them. Leave the herbs to soak for at least 15 minutes, or overnight.

2 Put the pot on the cooker. Bring the mixture to the boil, reduce to a simmer and cover. Cook for 30 minutes. Be careful not to let the herbs burn. Add more water if necessary.

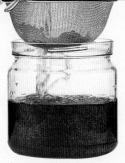

3 Strain the liquid into a container and put to one side. Leave the herbs in the cooking pot. Add more fresh water to the herbs in the pot, and cook for another 20 minutes.

4 Strain the liquid into the first batch of strained liquid. If there is too much sediment, you can strain the whole decoction again through a fine sieve or tea-strainer.

ESSENTIALS
Herbal decoctions are the traditional way of taking herbs.

—

The tastes and smells of Chinese herbal remedies may strike Western palates as strange to begin with.

Notes

- Do not take any other medicines within one hour of taking the herbs.
- Stop the herbs if you develop a full cold or flu.
- Stop the herbs if you have any unusual reactions or digestive upsets.
- Do not add sweeteners to the herbs as this will change their properties. A few drops of lemon juice on the tongue, after drinking the decoction, will take the taste away if required. For children, a little fruit juice can be added to the decoction.
- Take the herbs after food.
- The cooked herbs will keep in the fridge for up to a week.

Herbal formulas

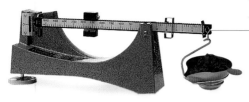

ABOVE **You will need scales capable of weighing small quantities, like these gunpowder scales.**

Chinese herbal formulas generally contain a main herb ('the emperor'), secondary herbs ('ministers') and herbs to add a directional quality to the mix ('assistants'). There is usually a 'harmonizer' to blend the mix into a remedy.

❶

STRENGTHEN EARTH DECOCTION

Ren Shen, 9g,
or Dang Shen, 18g
Bai Zhu, 12g
Fu Ling, 12g
Zhi Gan Cao, 6g
Yi Yi Ren, 9g
Chen Pi, 6g
Sha Ren, 6g
Lian Zi, 9g
Sheng Jiang, 6g

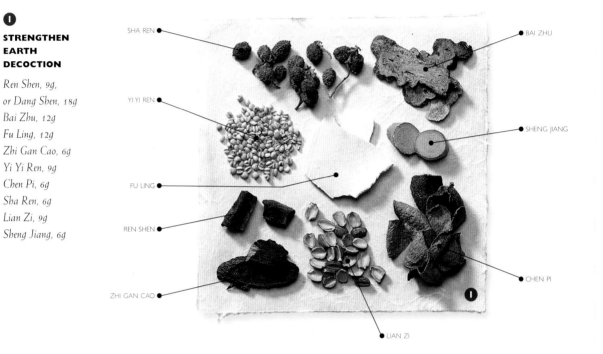

SHA REN
BAI ZHU
YI YI REN
SHENG JIANG
FU LING
REN SHEN
ZHI GAN CAO
CHEN PI
LIAN ZI

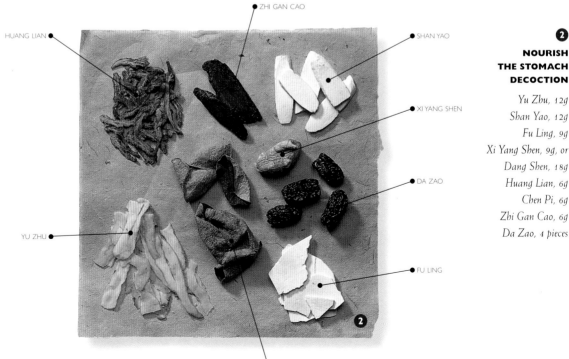

ZHI GAN CAO
HUANG LIAN
SHAN YAO
XI YANG SHEN
DA ZAO
YU ZHU
FU LING
CHEN PI

❷

NOURISH THE STOMACH DECOCTION

Yu Zhu, 12g
Shan Yao, 12g
Fu Ling, 9g
Xi Yang Shen, 9g, or
Dang Shen, 18g
Huang Lian, 6g
Chen Pi, 6g
Zhi Gan Cao, 6g
Da Zao, 4 pieces

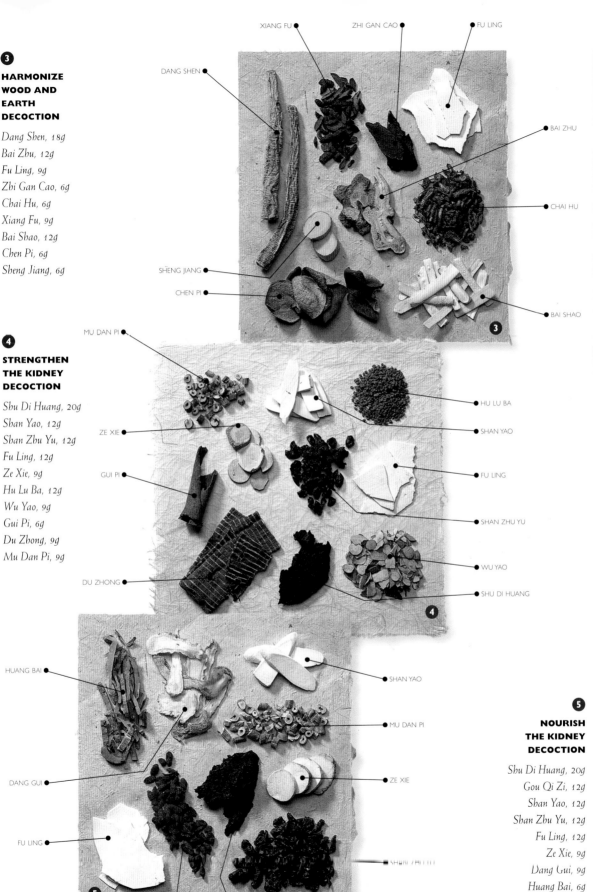

❸

HARMONIZE WOOD AND EARTH DECOCTION

Dang Shen, 18g
Bai Zhu, 12g
Fu Ling, 9g
Zhi Gan Cao, 6g
Chai Hu, 6g
Xiang Fu, 9g
Bai Shao, 12g
Chen Pi, 6g
Sheng Jiang, 6g

❹

STRENGTHEN THE KIDNEY DECOCTION

Shu Di Huang, 20g
Shan Yao, 12g
Shan Zhu Yu, 12g
Fu Ling, 12g
Ze Xie, 9g
Hu Lu Ba, 12g
Wu Yao, 9g
Gui Pi, 6g
Du Zhong, 9g
Mu Dan Pi, 9g

❺

NOURISH THE KIDNEY DECOCTION

Shu Di Huang, 20g
Gou Qi Zi, 12g
Shan Yao, 12g
Shan Zhu Yu, 12g
Fu Ling, 12g
Ze Xie, 9g
Dang Gui, 9g
Huang Bai, 6g
Mu Dan Pi, 9g

Labels on image ❸: XIANG FU, ZHI GAN CAO, FU LING, DANG SHEN, BAI ZHU, CHAI HU, SHENG JIANG, CHEN PI, BAI SHAO

Labels on image ❹: MU DAN PI, ZE XIE, GUI PI, DU ZHONG, HU LU BA, SHAN YAO, FU LING, SHAN ZHU YU, WU YAO, SHU DI HUANG

Labels on image ❺: HUANG BAI, DANG GUI, FU LING, SHAN YAO, MU DAN PI, ZE XIE, SHAN ZHU YU, GOU QI ZI, SHU DI HUANG

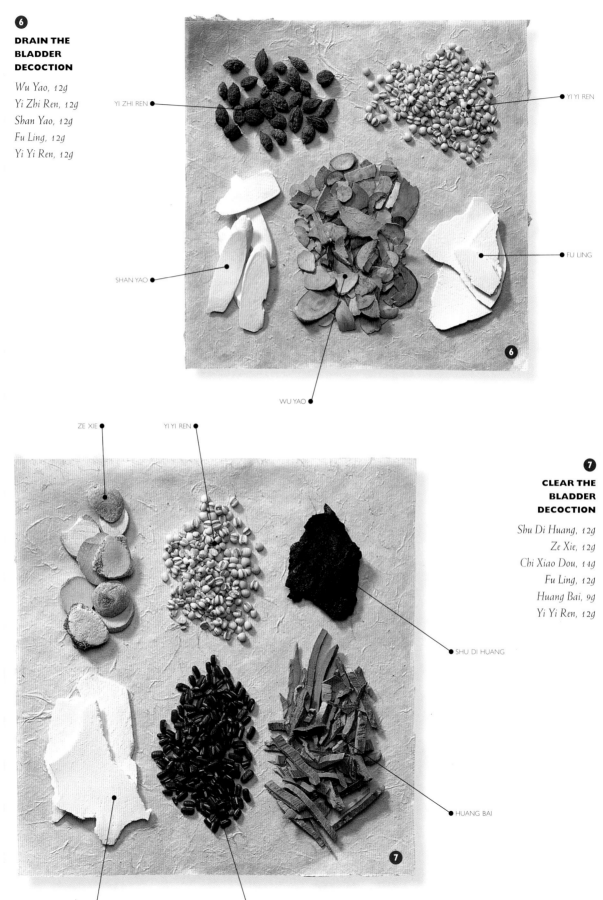

6

DRAIN THE BLADDER DECOCTION

Wu Yao, 12g
Yi Zhi Ren, 12g
Shan Yao, 12g
Fu Ling, 12g
Yi Yi Ren, 12g

YI ZHI REN

YI YI REN

SHAN YAO

FU LING

WU YAO

ZE XIE

YI YI REN

7

CLEAR THE BLADDER DECOCTION

Shu Di Huang, 12g
Ze Xie, 12g
Chi Xiao Dou, 14g
Fu Ling, 12g
Huang Bai, 9g
Yi Yi Ren, 12g

SHU DI HUANG

HUANG BAI

FU LING

CHI XIAO DOU

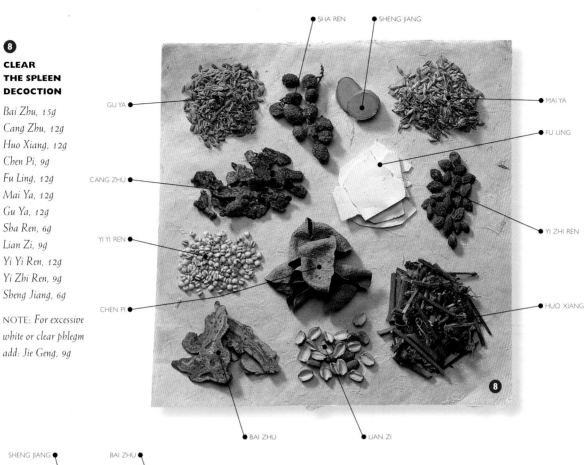

8

CLEAR THE SPLEEN DECOCTION

Bai Zhu, 15g
Cang Zhu, 12g
Huo Xiang, 12g
Chen Pi, 9g
Fu Ling, 12g
Mai Ya, 12g
Gu Ya, 12g
Sha Ren, 6g
Lian Zi, 9g
Yi Yi Ren, 12g
Yi Zhi Ren, 9g
Sheng Jiang, 6g

NOTE: *For excessive white or clear phlegm add: Jie Geng, 9g*

SHA REN · SHENG JIANG
GU YA ·
MAI YA ·
FU LING ·
CANG ZHU ·
YI ZHI REN ·
YI YI REN ·
CHEN PI ·
HUO XIANG ·
· BAI ZHU · LIAN ZI

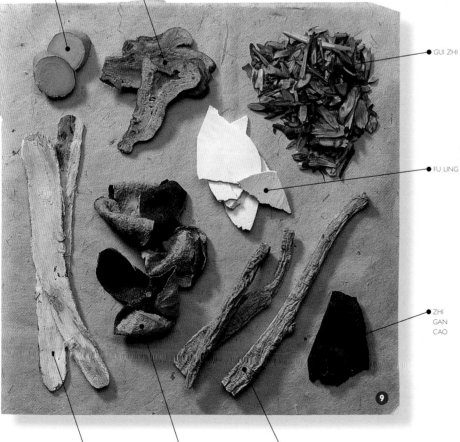

9

STRENGTHEN EARTH AND METAL DECOCTION

Huang Qi, 12g
Ren Shen, 9g, or
Dang Shen, 18g
Bai Zhu, 12g
Gui Zhi, 9g
Chen Pi, 6g
Fu Ling, 9g
Zhi Gan Cao, 6g
Sheng Jiang, 6g

NOTE: *To boost the immune system add: Ling Zhi, 9g, and Wu Wei Zi, 6g If there is wheezing add: Xing Ren, 6g For stuffy chest with catarrh add: Jie Geng, 9g For sneezing due to allergy add: Cang Er Zi, 9g*

SHENG JIANG · BAI ZHU ·
· GUI ZHI
· FU LING
· ZHI GAN CAO
· HUANG QI · CHEN PI · DANG SHEN

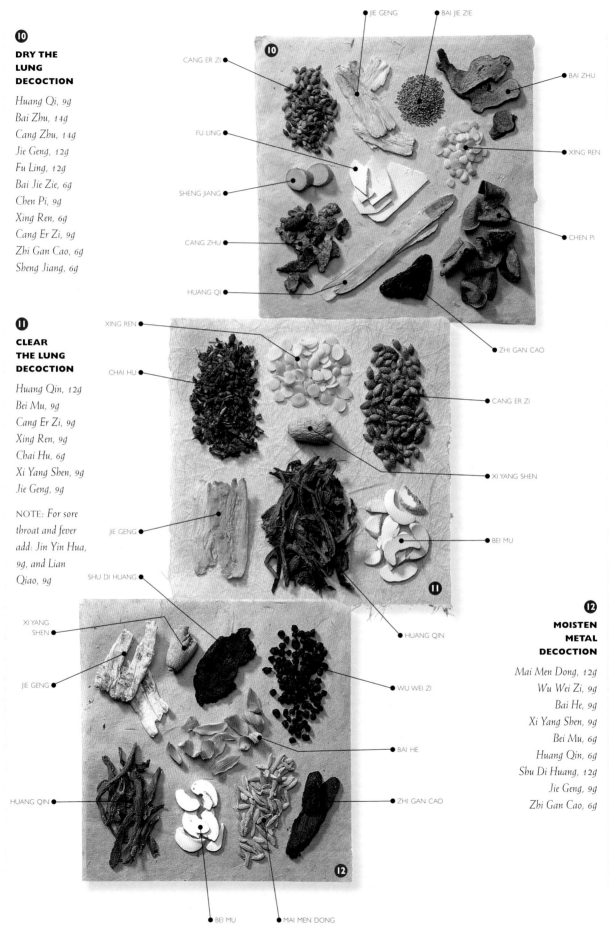

10

DRY THE LUNG DECOCTION

Huang Qi, 9g
Bai Zhu, 14g
Cang Zhu, 14g
Jie Geng, 12g
Fu Ling, 12g
Bai Jie Zie, 6g
Chen Pi, 9g
Xing Ren, 6g
Cang Er Zi, 9g
Zhi Gan Cao, 6g
Sheng Jiang, 6g

11

CLEAR THE LUNG DECOCTION

Huang Qin, 12g
Bei Mu, 9g
Cang Er Zi, 9g
Xing Ren, 9g
Chai Hu, 6g
Xi Yang Shen, 9g
Jie Geng, 9g

NOTE: *For sore throat and fever add: Jin Yin Hua, 9g, and Lian Qiao, 9g*

12

MOISTEN METAL DECOCTION

Mai Men Dong, 12g
Wu Wei Zi, 9g
Bai He, 9g
Xi Yang Shen, 9g
Bei Mu, 6g
Huang Qin, 6g
Shu Di Huang, 12g
Jie Geng, 9g
Zhi Gan Cao, 6g

Image 10 labels: JIE GENG, BAI JIE ZIE, CANG ER ZI, BAI ZHU, FU LING, XING REN, SHENG JIANG, CANG ZHU, CHEN PI, HUANG QI, ZHI GAN CAO

Image 11 labels: XING REN, CHAI HU, CANG ER ZI, XI YANG SHEN, JIE GENG, BEI MU, HUANG QIN

Image 12 labels: SHU DI HUANG, XI YANG SHEN, JIE GENG, WU WEI ZI, BAI HE, HUANG QIN, ZHI GAN CAO, BEI MU, MAI MEN DONG

13

NOURISH THE HEART DECOCTION

Ren Shen, 12g
Huang Qi, 12g
Dang Gui, 12g
Wu Wei Zi, 9g
Long Yan Rou, 9g
Zhi Gan Cao, 9g

NOTE: *When symptoms of Spleen Deficiency are also present add: Lian Zi, 9g, Bai Zhu, 12g, Fu Ling, 9g, Shan Zha, 9g*

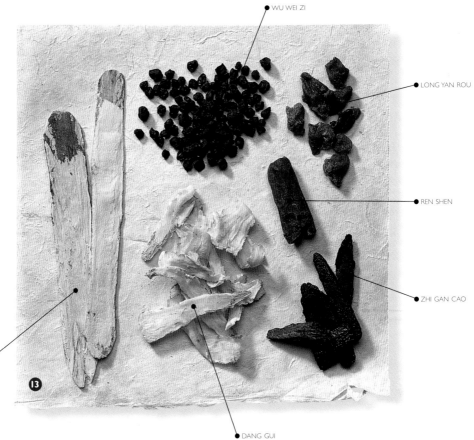

WU WEI ZI

LONG YAN ROU

REN SHEN

ZHI GAN CAO

HUANG QI

DANG GUI

14

NOURISH AND CALM THE HEART DECOCTION

Xi Yang Shen, 12g
Mai Men Dong, 12g
Huang Qin, 9g
Wu Wei Zi, 6g
Shu Di Huang, 12g
Fu Ling, 9g
Dang Shen, 6g
Suan Zao Ren, 9g
Yuan Zhi, 6g
Bai Zi Ren, 6g

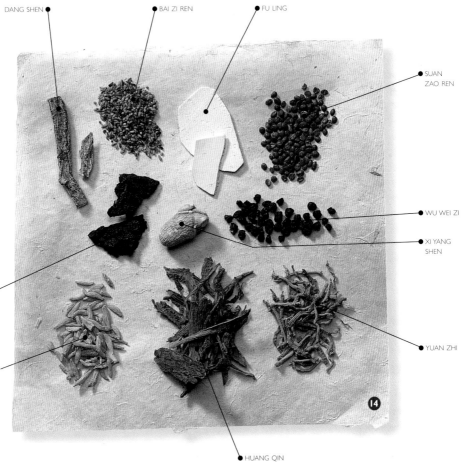

DANG SHEN

BAI ZI REN

FU LING

SUAN ZAO REN

WU WEI ZI

XI YANG SHEN

SHU DI HUANG

YUAN ZHI

MAI MEN DONG

HUANG QIN

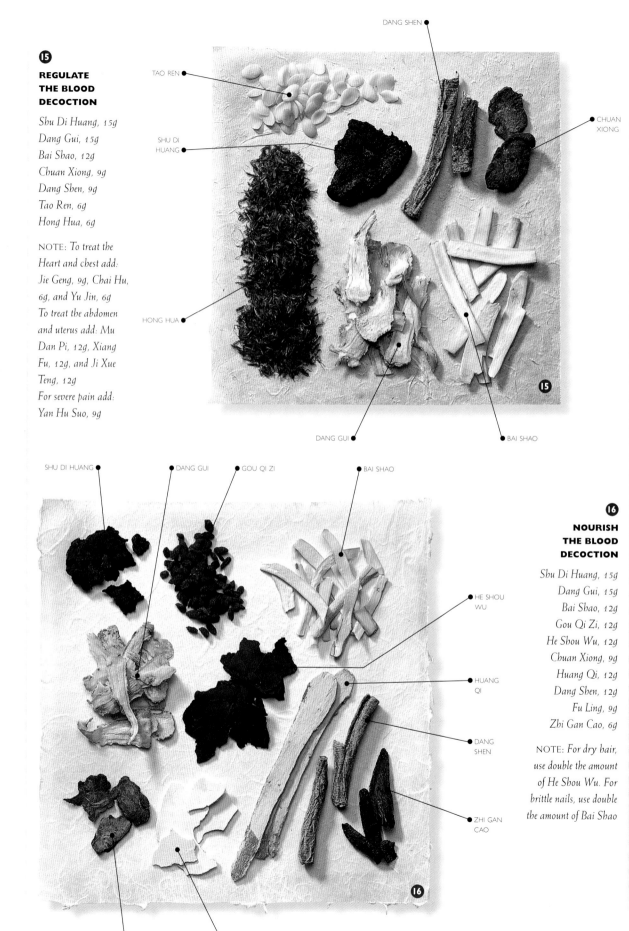

15

REGULATE THE BLOOD DECOCTION

Shu Di Huang, 15g

Dang Gui, 15g

Bai Shao, 12g

Chuan Xiong, 9g

Dang Shen, 9g

Tao Ren, 6g

Hong Hua, 6g

NOTE: *To treat the Heart and chest add: Jie Geng, 9g, Chai Hu, 6g, and Yu Jin, 6g To treat the abdomen and uterus add: Mu Dan Pi, 12g, Xiang Fu, 12g, and Ji Xue Teng, 12g For severe pain add: Yan Hu Suo, 9g*

DANG SHEN

TAO REN

SHU DI HUANG

CHUAN XIONG

HONG HUA

DANG GUI

BAI SHAO

SHU DI HUANG

DANG GUI

GOU QI ZI

BAI SHAO

HE SHOU WU

HUANG QI

DANG SHEN

ZHI GAN CAO

CHUAN XIONG

FU LING

16

NOURISH THE BLOOD DECOCTION

Shu Di Huang, 15g

Dang Gui, 15g

Bai Shao, 12g

Gou Qi Zi, 12g

He Shou Wu, 12g

Chuan Xiong, 9g

Huang Qi, 12g

Dang Shen, 12g

Fu Ling, 9g

Zhi Gan Cao, 6g

NOTE: *For dry hair, use double the amount of He Shou Wu. For brittle nails, use double the amount of Bai Shao*

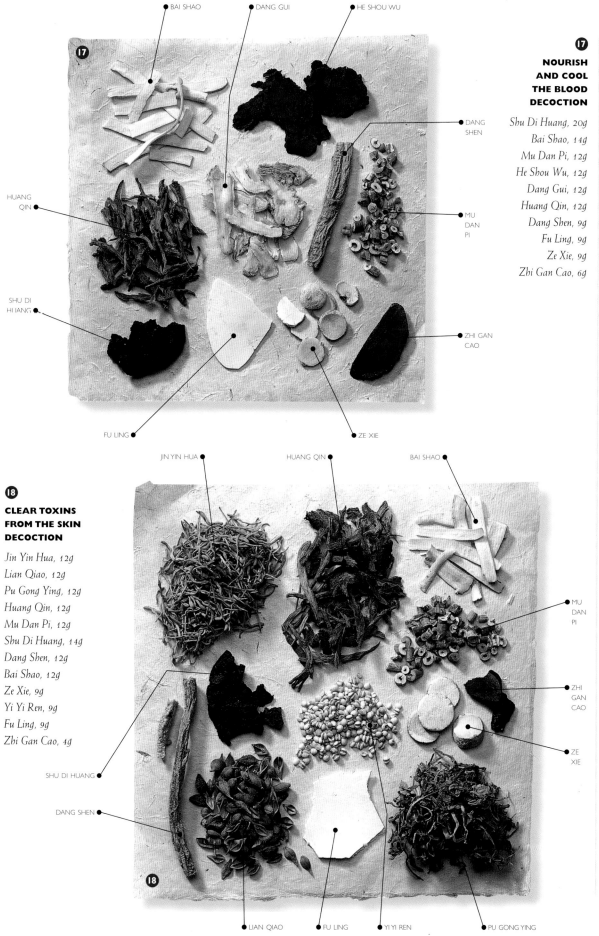

BAI SHAO

DANG GUI

HE SHOU WU

17

17

NOURISH AND COOL THE BLOOD DECOCTION

Shu Di Huang, 20g

Bai Shao, 14g

Mu Dan Pi, 12g

He Shou Wu, 12g

Dang Gui, 12g

Huang Qin, 12g

Dang Shen, 9g

Fu Ling, 9g

Ze Xie, 9g

Zhi Gan Cao, 6g

DANG SHEN

HUANG QIN

MU DAN PI

SHU DI HUANG

ZHI GAN CAO

FU LING

ZE XIE

JIN YIN HUA

HUANG QIN

BAI SHAO

18

CLEAR TOXINS FROM THE SKIN DECOCTION

Jin Yin Hua, 12g

Lian Qiao, 12g

Pu Gong Ying, 12g

Huang Qin, 12g

Mu Dan Pi, 12g

Shu Di Huang, 14g

Dang Shen, 12g

Bai Shao, 12g

Ze Xie, 9g

Yi Yi Ren, 9g

Fu Ling, 9g

Zhi Gan Cao, 4g

MU DAN PI

ZHI GAN CAO

ZE XIE

SHU DI HUANG

DANG SHEN

18

LIAN QIAO

FU LING

YI YI REN

PU GONG YING

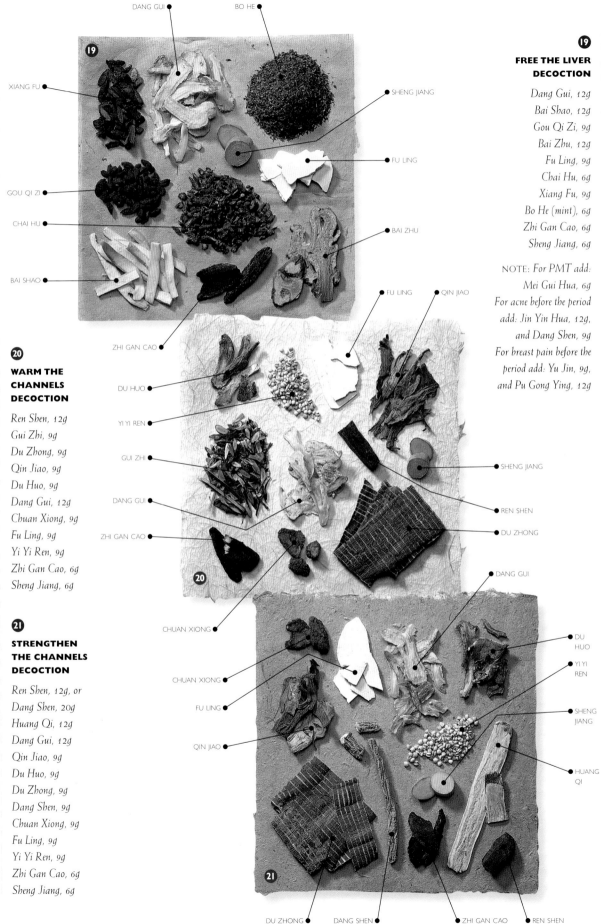

DANG GUI

BO HE

19

XIANG FU

SHENG JIANG

FU LING

GOU QI ZI

CHAI HU

BAI ZHU

BAI SHAO

ZHI GAN CAO

FU LING

QIN JIAO

19

FREE THE LIVER DECOCTION

Dang Gui, 12g

Bai Shao, 12g

Gou Qi Zi, 9g

Bai Zhu, 12g

Fu Ling, 9g

Chai Hu, 6g

Xiang Fu, 9g

Bo He (mint), 6g

Zhi Gan Cao, 6g

Sheng Jiang, 6g

NOTE: *For PMT add:*
Mei Gui Hua, 6g
For acne before the period
add: Jin Yin Hua, 12g,
and Dang Shen, 9g
For breast pain before the
period add: Yu Jin, 9g,
and Pu Gong Ying, 12g

20

WARM THE CHANNELS DECOCTION

Ren Shen, 12g

Gui Zhi, 9g

Du Zhong, 9g

Qin Jiao, 9g

Du Huo, 9g

Dang Gui, 12g

Chuan Xiong, 9g

Fu Ling, 9g

Yi Yi Ren, 9g

Zhi Gan Cao, 6g

Sheng Jiang, 6g

DU HUO

YI YI REN

GUI ZHI

DANG GUI

ZHI GAN CAO

SHENG JIANG

REN SHEN

DU ZHONG

20

DANG GUI

CHUAN XIONG

21

STRENGTHEN THE CHANNELS DECOCTION

Ren Shen, 12g, or
Dang Shen, 20g

Huang Qi, 12g

Dang Gui, 12g

Qin Jiao, 9g

Du Huo, 9g

Du Zhong, 9g

Dang Shen, 9g

Chuan Xiong, 9g

Fu Ling, 9g

Yi Yi Ren, 9g

Zhi Gan Cao, 6g

Sheng Jiang, 6g

CHUAN XIONG

FU LING

QIN JIAO

DU HUO

YI YI REN

SHENG JIANG

HUANG QI

21

DU ZHONG

DANG SHEN

ZHI GAN CAO

REN SHEN

22

AID THE YOUNG DIGESTION DECOCTION

Dang Shen, 9g
Bai Zhu, 9g
Fu Ling, 9g
Zhi Gan Cao, 6g
Chen Pi, 4g
Jie Geng, 6g
Yi Yi Ren, 6g
Shan Zha, 6g
Mai Ya, 6g
Gu Ya, 6g
Shen Qu, 6g
Sheng Jiang, 4g

NOTE: *the dosage given here is the 'adult' dose for older children of around fourteen. It should be reduced according to the ratios given on page 89 for younger children and babies.*

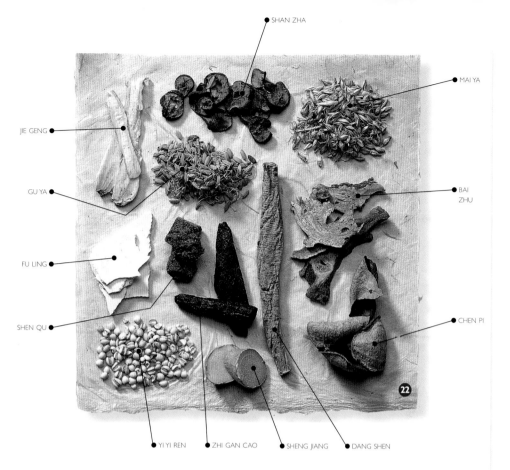

SHAN ZHA
JIE GENG
GU YA
FU LING
SHEN QU
MAI YA
BAI ZHU
CHEN PI
YI YI REN
ZHI GAN CAO
SHENG JIANG
DANG SHEN

23

STRENGTHEN THE QI IN THE YOUNG DECOCTION

Dang Shen, 12g
Bai Zhu, 9g
Huang Qi, 12g
Fu Ling, 9g
Sha Ren, 3g
Gui Zhi, 6g
Wu Wei Zi, 6g
Mai Ya, 6g
Gu Ya, 6g
Shen Qu, 6g
Shan Zha, 6g
Zhi Gan Cao, 6g

NOTE: *the dosage given here is the 'adult' dose for older children of around fourteen. It should be reduced according to the ratios given on page 89 for younger children and babies.*

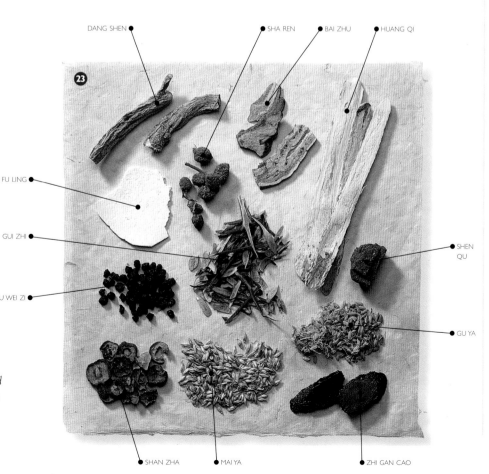

DANG SHEN
SHA REN
BAI ZHU
HUANG QI
FU LING
GUI ZHI
SHEN QU
WU WEI ZI
GU YA
SHAN ZHA
MAI YA
ZHI GAN CAO

FOOD

Foods are classified in exactly the same way as herbs. Each food has a temperature, a taste and one or several organ systems that it affects. The concept of food therapy is a huge one: here is a taster, with recipes for each season or Element. These meals can be eaten as a seasonal balancing agent.

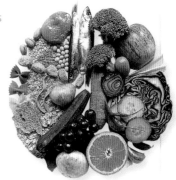

ABOVE **Certain foods – fresh fruit and vegetables, and lean fish – provide a daily programme of health maintenance.**

Recipes

SUMMER SOLSTICE SALAD WITH GRILLED VEGETABLES
Fire Element

—

INGREDIENTS
2 medium carrots
quarter of a white cabbage
1 small mooli or daikon radish
half a celeriac head
1 large scallion
2 tblsp toasted sesame or hemp seeds
juice of half a medium lemon or a whole lime
1 sweet red pepper
4 shallots or 1 large red onion
1 small fennel bulb
4 cloves garlic with the skin left on
6 tblsp olive oil
1 tblsp toasted sesame oil or hemp oil

🌿 Core and quarter the pepper, peel the onion (or shallots) and slice the fennel. Put in an oven dish, together with the garlic, and cover with the olive oil. Place under the grill for 20 minutes, until soft.
🌿 For the salad, shred the carrot, cabbage, mooli and celeriac. Slice the scallion and add, along with the seeds. Season and mix with the citrus juice.

🌿 Spoon the grilled vegetables on to the salad, and then pour the warm oil from the oven dish over the top. Add the sesame oil and serve immediately as a starter or side dish. Serves four.

ORANGE-ROASTED VEGETABLES
Earth Element

—

INGREDIENTS
1 large onion, cut into 8 pieces
2 large unpeeled carrots, cut into chunks
8 cloves unpeeled garlic
2 celery stalks, cut into chunks
1 small broccoli, cut into florets
half a small squash or pumpkin, cubed
1 orange, quartered
dried herbs such as bay leaf, rosemary or oregano
150ml (¼pt /⅔ cup) olive oil

🌿 Place all the vegetables and dried herbs in an oven dish and cover with the oil. Squeeze the juice from the orange segments over the vegetables. Put the segments to roast with the rest of the ingredients.
🌿 Bake uncovered in a pre-heated medium oven 180°C/350°F/gas 4 for 45 minutes, turning once or twice. The water in the vegetables will come out as they are cooked, and they will be steam-roasted.
🌿 Serve in a warmed dish, spooning some of the oil from the oven dish over the vegetables. Season with sea salt, pepper and kelp flakes.
🌿 Eat as a main course (ideally with rice that has been boiled with safflower or a few strands of saffron to give it an orange colour), or as a vegetable dish with fish or meat. Serves four.

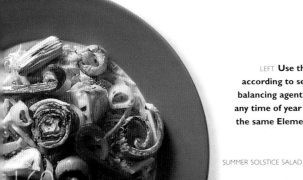

LEFT **Use the recipes according to season as a balancing agent, or eat at any time of year if you are the same Elemental type.**

AROMATIC AUTUMN NUT FEAST
Metal Element

▬

INGREDIENTS

FOR THE NUT FEAST
450g (1lb /3½ cups) mixed nuts and seeds (e.g. brazils, cashews,
almonds, sesame seeds, sunflower seeds)
4 cloves garlic
1 egg or 2 tblsp whey powder
250ml (8fl.oz /1 cup) milk (rice or sheep's)
50g (2oz /1 cup) fresh breadcrumbs, or 100g (4oz /1 cup)
stuffing mix
1 tsp each of ginger powder, crushed cardamom and black pepper
sea salt
olive oil and water

FOR THE TOMATO MOLÉ
tin of plum tomatoes
tin of pimentos (optional)
½ tsp each of spices such as cayenne pepper, turmeric, allspice
and nutmeg
1 tblsp honey vinegar
1 tblsp wine vinegar

❧ Crush the nuts, seeds and garlic.

❧ Mix in all the other ingredients, adding enough oil and water to bind them into a thick paste. Spoon into a greased, deep-sided baking dish. Bake uncovered in a medium oven 180°C/350°F/gas 4 for 45 minutes, until the top is golden brown.

❧ To make the tomato molé, liquidize the tomatoes (and pimentos) in a blender and strain through a fine sieve to remove the seeds. Warm in a heavy pan, and add the spices. Cover the molé and put aside until required. Just before serving, heat it up again and stir in the honey and wine vinegars.

❧ Serve slices of the nut feast on top of a layer of the spicy tomato molé, with a green salad. Serves four.

LIVE SPRING SALAD
Wood Element

▬

SALAD INGREDIENTS
350g (12oz /3 cups) fresh
sprouted pulses, thoroughly rinsed
100g (4oz /1 cup) alfalfa
sprouts, rinsed and chopped
100g (4oz /1 cup) mixed
sunflower and sesame seeds
(and hemp seeds if available)

FOR THE DRESSING
150ml (¼pt /½ cup) mixed oils
(olive, sesame,
walnut, flax or hemp)
1 tsp light soy sauce (or liquid aminos)
2 tblsp tahini (sesame paste)
1 or 2 cloves garlic, crushed
1 or 2 tblsp balsamic, wine or rice vinegar
(lemon juice can be substituted)
1 tblsp kelp flakes
1 tsp grain mustard or horseradish
black pepper to taste

❧ Blend the dressing ingredients together. Mix all the salad ingredients in a bowl, and toss with the dressing.

❧ Serve the salad as a side dish, or with soba or buckwheat noodles that have been cooked and then refreshed in cold water. Serves four.

WINTER BROTH
Water Element

▬

INGREDIENTS
1 leek, sliced
1 or 2 onions, finely sliced
3 sticks celery, diced
2 medium carrots, diced
1 small cabbage, chopped
a strip of kombu seaweed
(around 15cm /6in long)
100g (4oz /½ cup) wholegrain barley
100g (4oz /½ cup) yellow split peas, soaked
600ml (1pt /2½ cups) vegetable or
chicken stock
50g (2oz /½ cup) chopped parsley
Miso to taste (around 1 tblsp)
1–2l (2–3 pt /5–10 cups) water
black pepper

WINTER
BROTH

❧ Gently soften the vegetables with a little olive oil over a low heat.

❧ Fill a large cooking pot with the water, add the split peas, barley and kombu. Bring to the boil, reduce the heat to a simmer, and cook for half an hour.

❧ Add the vegetables, stock and parsley, and simmer for another 20–30 minutes. Dilute the miso with some warm water and add for the last five minutes.

❧ Season with the black pepper and serve straight away, with fresh crusty rye bread or oat cakes. This hearty soup serves four.

MEDICINAL WINES

There is a long tradition of taking herbs as 'tonic wines' in the East, particularly where expensive herbs are involved. Wines are often used during recovery from illness. The alcohol should be regarded as an integral ingredient in these tonic formulas and its action taken into account. Alcohol is warming and invigorating, moves the Qi and Blood, and activates the Yang energy.

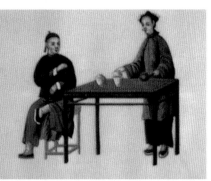

ABOVE **Herbal tonic wines are enjoyable medicaments, and have long been used in China.**

Alcohol power

The properties of alcohol can be used to great advantage where there is Internal Cold or Yang Deficiency, or where there is pain due to Blood Stasis. However, care should obviously be taken if the patient has too much Heat in the body, or is a recovering alcoholic.

Traditionally, rice wine, or Jiu (pronounced 'jew'), is used, but for taste and convenience we in the West can substitute spirits. I generally prefer vodka as it is neutral in taste, but gin or brandy are also suitable. Saké can be used if you want a more traditional formula.

RIGHT **Alcohol preserves the potency of herbs in a convenient form, and is seen as a beneficial ingredient in its own right.**

ESSENTIALS

Alcohol warms and strengthens Yang energies, and so makes a useful base for certain remedies.

—

Different herbs can be used in the wines to counter specific health problems.

Making a medicinal wine

The procedure for making any of these special elixirs is essentially the same. All the formulas are based on using 500ml (¾pt /2 cups) of alcohol.

1 Break the herbs into small pieces and place them in a lidded jar or similar sealable container.

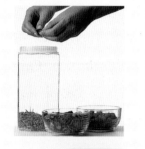

2 Add the alcohol. Leave the mixture for two to three weeks. Gently shake the mixture once or twice a week during this period.

3 Strain the liquid through a fine sieve and put into bottles.

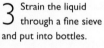

DOSAGE

Generally, one has a 'wee dram' of the wine each day if it is being taken as a general tonic, or as required if being taken for a specific purpose.

NOTE FOR REN SHEN HUANG QI JIN
Ginseng is expensive, so do not crush the herbs in this formula. Leave the wine for one month, then discard the Huang Qi before drinking. When it is finished, add fresh Huang Qi and alcohol to make a new batch. (This will not be as strong.)

DANG GUI BAI SHAO JIU
ANGELICA AND PEONY WINE

Dang Gui, 100g	Chuan Xiong, 50g
Bai Shao, 100g	Xiang Fu, 50g

ACTION

For irregular periods and mood swings.

REN SHEN HUANG QI JIU
GINSENG AND ASTRAGALUS WINE

Ren Shen, 50g
Huang Qi, 100g

ACTION

Strengthens Qi and immunity. See note below left.

HONG HUA DANG GUI JIU
SAFFLOWER AND ANGELICA WINE

Hong Hua, 100g
Dang Gui, 200g

ACTION

For painful and irregular periods.

BU ZHONG JIU
BOOST THE MIDDLE WINE

Hui Xiang, 50g
Shan Zha, 100g
Sha Ren, 50g

ACTION

Strengthens and warms the digestion when there is poor appetite, nausea, bloating and dull stomach pain. Take before or after food to assist digestion.

BU XU JIU
FILL EMPTINESS WINE

Dang Gui, 50g	Wu Wei Zi, 30g
Bai Shao, 40g	Shan Yao, 50g
Long Yan Rou, 50g	Du Zhong, 50g
Ren Shen, 50g	Zhi Gan Cao, 25g
Gou Qi Zi, 50g	

ACTION

Restores vitality after a long illness or childbirth.

GUI XIONG JIU
CINNAMON AND LIGUSTICUM WINE

Du Zhong, 100g	Chuan Xiong, 50g
Qin Jiao, 50g	Gui Zhi, 30g
Du Huo, 50g	

ACTION

For pain and stiffness in the back, legs and knees, which is worse in cold and damp weather.

CREAMS AND OINTMENTS

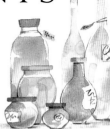

Herbal preparations can also be used on the body. Crushed herbs, in a poultice, deliver a strong dose of the remedy to a specific area. You can also make lotions based on tinctures or infusions, or creams to soften the skin.

TINCTURE TO STRENGTHEN THE HAIR

This tincture is used to keep the hair and scalp in a healthy condition, and can be helpful if the hair is thinning or there is dandruff.

Chuan Xiong, 50g	*Dan Shen,* 50g
He Shou Wu, 50g	*Bai Shao,* 50g
Sheng Jiang, 50g	

✍ Break the herbs up into small pieces and place in a jar with 500ml (¾pt /2 cups) of pure spirit such as vodka. After two weeks, strain off the spirit through a fine sieve and keep in a bottle.

✍ Pour about two tablespoonsful of the liquid on to the scalp and massage in vigorously with the finger-tips. Leave in for at least fifteen minutes (up to an hour), then wash and condition the hair. The tincture can be used up to twice a week, as required.

MASSAGE VIGOROUSLY ●

TINCTURE TO WARM THE CHANNELS

People with poor circulation can be very sensitive to the cold. This tincture can be used on the hands in cold weather as an alcohol rub.

Dang Gui, 50g	*Sheng Jiang,* 50g
Hong Hua, 30g	*Hu Jiao,* 30g
Gui Zhi, 60g	*Zhang Nao,* 15g

✍ Break all the herbs into small pieces and place in a jar with 500ml (¾pt /2 cups) of pure spirit such as vodka. Strain the liquid off into bottles after one week and label 'for external use only'.

✍ Pour some of the tincture on to your hands and rub in until dry. Use as required.

NOTE: Zhang Nao is camphor, which can be obtained in blocks from most chemists. It is a toxic substance and must not be taken internally.

FACIAL WASH TO CLEANSE THE SKIN

The mixture of herbs blended together in this facial wash has detoxifying and antiviral properties, and can be used for spots and irritated skin.

Jin Yin Hua, 20g	*Ju Hua,* 20g
Pu Gong Ying, 20g	*Huang Qing,* 30g

✍ Add all the herbs to a pot with 600ml (1pt /2½cups) of water and leave to soak for a few minutes. Bring to the boil and then simmer gently for 20–30 minutes. Strain, cool, then bottle. Keep in the fridge and discard after a week.

✍ Wash the face or the affected part with the cleansing solution last thing at night, and leave the solution on overnight. The next morning, the skin should be rinsed thoroughly with fresh water. Can be used once or twice a week, as required.

LEFT **Hair and scalp problems respond to tincture use.**

COLD-SORE PASTE

Cold sores can be painful and unsightly. This soothing paste can be used for herpes outbreaks on any part of the body, not just the face.

❙ *Huang Lian, 20g*

🌿 Powder the herb finely and mix into a paste with a small amount of fresh plantain (banana can be used if this is not available). Store in a salad jar in the fridge. It will keep for about a week.

🌿 Cover the affected area with the paste and leave on for as long as possible. Repeat as necessary.

EYEBATH INFUSION

Redness and itching of the eyes may result from hay fever, pollution, or spending too long working on a computer. Ju Hua (chrysanthemum) is a traditional remedy for cooling and brightening the eyes, whether used internally or as an eyewash.

❙ *Ju Hua, 5g*

🌿 Put the flowers in a bowl and pour on boiling water. Leave to infuse for ten to fifteen minutes and then strain carefully. Use when cool. Store in the fridge and use within two days.

🌿 Use as an eyebath when required. If treating both eyes, remember to wash the eyebath well in between to avoid the risk of cross-contamination.

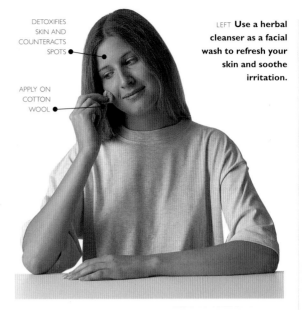

DETOXIFIES SKIN AND COUNTERACTS SPOTS

APPLY ON COTTON WOOL

LEFT Use a herbal cleanser as a facial wash to refresh your skin and soothe irritation.

SKIN-TONING CREAM

There is an increasing trend in the cosmetics industry towards using herbs and other natural substances in beauty products. Here is a recipe you can easily make up for yourself, which contains several of the most effective toning ingredients.

Ren Shen, 20g **❙**
He Shou Wu, 20g **❙**
Qing Cha, 10g **❙**
(green tea)

❙ *Lu Hui (Aloe Vera liquid), 20ml (2 tblsp)*
❙ *Aqueous cream, 250ml (8fl.oz /1 cup). This is available from any chemist*

🌿 Break the Ren Shen, He Shou Wu and Qing Cha into small pieces and put in a pot with 600ml (1pt /2½ cups) of water. Bring to the boil and then reduce heat to a simmer. Cook with the lid on until the liquid is reduced to about half a cup, and then strain into a bowl. When cool, mix in the aqueous cream and Lu Hui. Stir the mixture thoroughly to stop the oils and water in the cream from separating and to ensure the mix is well blended. Store in an airtight jar and keep in the fridge.

🌿 Use on the face as a night cream and clean off in the morning.

BELOW **An infusion of chrysanthemum soothes tired and irritated eyes.**

RIGHT **Skin-toning cream contains green tea, which has an antioxidant action.**

CHRYSANTHEMUM PETALS

APPLY BEFORE BED

ESSENTIALS
Most applications will keep for a few days. Store in the fridge.

Strain mixtures thoroughly, especially when making eyebaths.

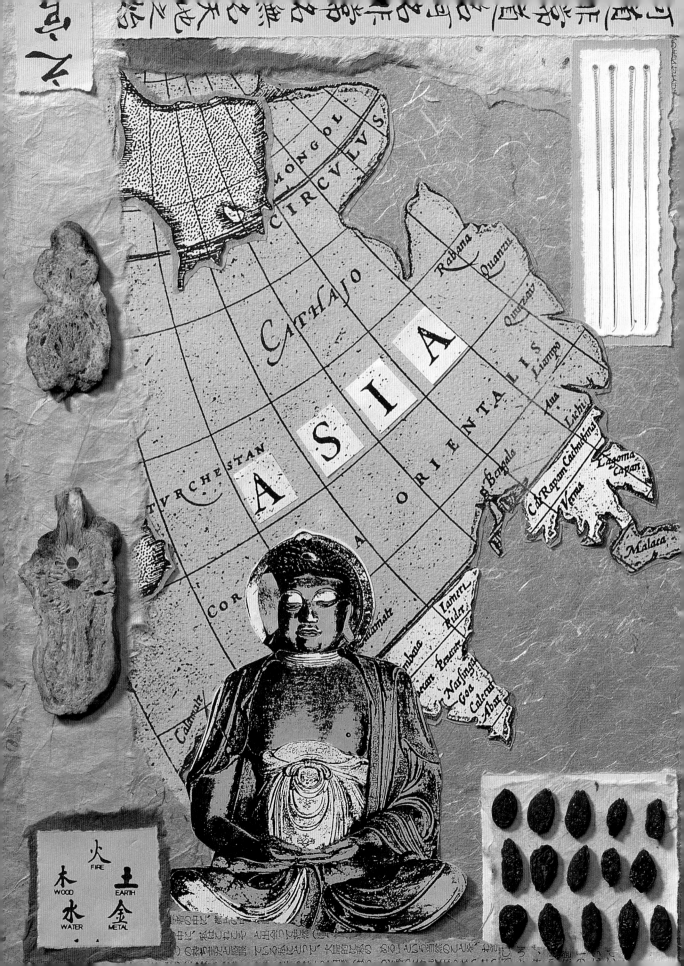

PART FIVE

YOUR GOOD HEALTH

This book is designed as a source of practical information, and Part Five also includes strategies for maintaining health in the face of the challenges presented by modern life. However, no book on Chinese Medicine would be complete without an overview of the background to this fascinating subject, so read on to find out more about its origins and influences. This section also tells you what you can expect when you consult a Chinese herbalist, and how to find a good practitioner.

膻中者

THE HISTORY OF ORIENTAL MEDICINE

Two important figures are at the root of Chinese Medicine. The Yellow Emperor (Huang Di) – the 'Divine Centre of the universe' – lends his name to the earliest major book, the Classic of Internal Medicine of the Yellow Emperor (Huang Di Nei Jing). It takes the form of conversations between the Yellow Emperor and his physician, Qi Bo.

SHEN NONG

In China, philosophy and medicine have always been inseparable, and it is from legend that the organized system of Chinese medicine first emerges.

One such figure of legend is Shen Nong, the Divine Farmer. Shen Nong was also known as the Fire or Red Emperor, and he is said to have taught mankind to grow food and herbs. The Divine Farmer possessed a magical ability to work out the properties of plants and herbs, which he would then test by eating the plants himself. Because of his power, he could even ingest poisonous plants without harm. However, one day he overstretched his body's ability to neutralize poisons, and died. The results of his studies were collected in the *Divine Farmer's Classic of Herbal Medicine (Shen Nong Ben Cao Jing)*, a list of all the important herbs and their properties.

I CHING

The *I Ching* (or *Yi Jing*, the *Classic of Change*), has been used by many people in the West as a kind of fortune-telling device, rather like tarot cards. Although this is one of the book's applications, this is not its most important contribution. The *I Ching* is the classic Taoist text and introduced the concept of Yin and Yang for the first time, in the form of the solid and broken lines that make up trigrams and hexagrams throughout the book. The idea is that an apparently randomly generated pattern can reveal the answer to any question directed at it, as long as you have the knowledge to interpret the result.

The first versions of the *I Ching* probably date back to the Hsia Dynasty (2205–1766 BC). Later, the philosopher Confucius did much to codify the work, a task that was continued by his disciples.

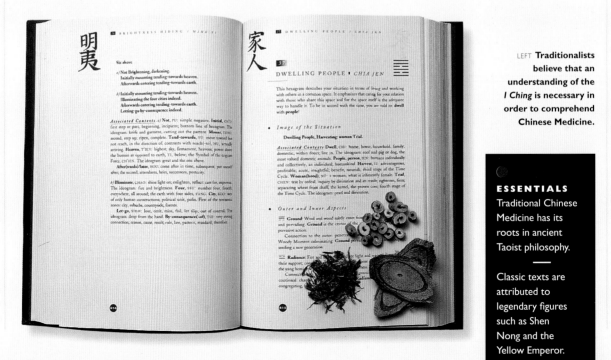

LEFT **Traditionalists believe that an understanding of the *I Ching* is necessary in order to comprehend Chinese Medicine.**

ESSENTIALS

Traditional Chinese Medicine has its roots in ancient Taoist philosophy.

—

Classic texts are attributed to legendary figures such as Shen Nong and the Yellow Emperor.

MODERN DEVELOPMENTS

It was not until President Nixon's historic visit to China in the early 1970s that acupuncture became known to many people in the West. Since then there has been a steady increase in the level of interest in, and the availability of, Chinese Medicine. Millions of people have now received the benefit of traditional treatment. But because our introduction to the tradition was through acupuncture, this is perhaps still better known than herbalism.

HERBS VERSUS ACUPUNCTURE

In China, herbal medicine has always been the main method of treating illness. Acupuncture was mostly practised by scholars who treated the top end of the social hierarchy. Folk doctors could perform basic acupuncture treatment, but this was not at the advanced level of the scholar doctor. Most people consulted the local herbalist if they were ill.

In the West, most people's only knowledge of Chinese Medicine is an awareness of acupuncture. There are many acupuncturists practising their craft. It is only in the last few years, with the opening up of Chinese society, that herbal medicine is assuming its rightful place as the mainstay of the Chinese system of medicine.

Most herbalists are also acupuncturists, but an acupuncturist won't necessarily have a knowledge of herbs. Although the diagnostic and theoretical background come from the same root, the practice of herbal medicine is a special and unique tradition within China.

HERBAL MEDICINE IS BECOMING BETTER KNOWN IN THE WEST

HERBALISM HAS ALWAYS BEEN THE BEST-KNOWN MEDICINE SYSTEM IN CHINA

ACUPUNCTURE IS A MINORITY TREATMENT IN CHINA BUT IS WELL KNOWN IN THE WEST

ABOVE **Herbalism and acupuncture have spread from their Eastern origins to a Western audience.**

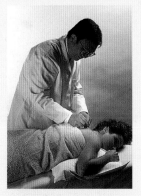

LEFT **Acupuncture involves stimulating various points on the Meridians.**

TRADITIONAL CHINESE MEDICINE

Chairman Mao Tse Dong standardized all the different medical traditions into a system called Traditional Chinese Medicine (TCM). But during Mao's Cultural Revolution, much traditional knowledge was lost. Now some of it is beginning to surface in the West: we seem to be more interested in it than people are in China, where modern science is being rigorously applied to TCM. This is only in keeping with Yin and Yang: as the East becomes a more dominant Yang culture, it is the West that probably represents the future of the ideas behind Chinese Medicine.

FENG SHUI

Archaeological evidence shows that Feng Shui has been practised in China for about 2,000 years. Literally translated, Feng means 'wind' and Shui means 'water', but this gives little insight into the broad applications of the science. A better translation might be 'environment', as Feng Shui is concerned with understanding the properties of universal energy (Qi), and using it to create places to live that have auspicious effects on the inhabitants' lives.

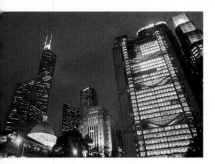

ABOVE **Some businesses apply Feng Shui rules to the planning of their offices.**

Consulting a master

The early Feng Shui master's job was to look at the natural features of a location and determine the right places for business, fortifications, creativity and rest. His tools included a compass, dowsing rods and probably a copy of the *Li Shu (Book of Rights)*, a sacred book expounding the tenets of Chinese religious belief. Knowledge of the rich symbolism of Chinese philosophy, religion and culture increased his experience.

INGRAINED VALUES

The first book on Feng Shui was written in the ninth century. Not only buildings but whole landscapes were affected: rivers were diverted and hills reshaped to improve the fortunes of the emperor. The basic principles of Feng Shui were second nature to the Chinese, but an acknowledgement of the master's art and the limited writing on the subject meant that people would always consult a practitioner before building. Feng Shui was closely woven into the disciplines of architecture, surveying, building and interior design, and Feng Shui masters would automatically be involved in

SMALL BUILDINGS WITH TALLER NEIGHBOURS HAVE BAD FENG SHUI

TREES OBSCURE SUNLIGHT: CUT THEM BACK

ABOVE **Modern towns and cities present a challenge for Feng Shui: there are many negative aspects to overcome.**

QI ACCUMULATES IN WATER, MAKING RIVERSIDE SITES VERY AUSPICIOUS

SLOW, MEANDERING RIVERS BRING GOOD LUCK

any new construction project. Even a ban on it during the Cultural Revolution, though it might have put Feng Shui masters out of work, had very little effect on its practical application. Ironically, the decision to ban the practice of Feng Shui would probably have been taken in a room perfectly sited for power!

Doors and windows

Doors and windows are seen as the mouth and eyes of the house, allowing the right amount of Qi to enter; however it can easily flow out of the house the same way. Stairs leading directly to the front door are seen as particularly unlucky, as good fortune simply runs down the staircase and away. Hanging wind chimes, or placing a mirror behind the door, will help to deflect the Qi and keep good luck inside. Interior doors help to pump Qi around the house and should open into a room. Hanging mirrors on adjacent walls will help to catch the Qi.

Outward or inward opening windows are preferred to those that slide up and down, because they allow the most Qi to flow into the home. Hanging crystal balls in windows that face west is another Feng Shui tactic – it converts the bright afternoon glare into a myriad of lucky colours, vitalizing the room with Qi.

BUILDIINGS WHICH FACE A PARK OR GARDEN ENJOY GOOD FENG SHUI

FENG SHUI TAKES ALL ASPECTS OF THE LANDSCAPE INTO CONSIDERATION

HOUSES WHICH FACE ROADS ARE AUSPICIOUS – THE ROAD BRINGS QI STRAIGHT TO THEIR FRONT DOORS

ESSENTIALS
Feng Shui is about harmonizing our interaction with the environment, using simple tactics to ensure a beneficial energy flow.

The principles of Feng Shui have been practised for about 2,000 years.

MODERN FENG SHUI

In the ninth century, the various schools of Feng Shui were broadly grouped into two categories. These were the form school (studying the scenic configurations of the land) and the compass school (focusing on the technical and scientific application of the compass). These are the classic schools: various aspects of each have been combined in a simplified system of Feng Shui which is now widely practised in the West. This system does not use the precision of the compass but simply the Ba Gua – a nine-square grid in which each square represents an aspect of life (e.g. relationships, wealth, blessings). This is placed over a plan of your home, or each room. Areas that are inauspicious can then be enhanced, and if there is too much energy in an area, it can be minimized.

APPLYING THE PRINCIPLES

In simple terms, everything about your home (from its location and layout, to where you put your grandfather clock) can have a powerful positive or negative effect on every aspect of your life. The ideal house would be built from scratch in a great location, designed along smooth lines to aid the flow of energy. Each room would be sited according to its function.

In reality, though, most of us move into an existing house complete with windows, doors and walls in fixed positions, and maybe a telegraph pole outside the bedroom window and an underground stream running directly beneath the kitchen. Reducing negative effects like these gives Feng Shui its biggest challenge. A compass is used to apply the principles of the Five Elements to the building and each room. Energy is then balanced with colour, plants, crystals, water, wind chimes and more.

WHAT ARE WE LOOKING FOR?

Profound effects on health, wealth and fulfilment are routinely reported in the many hundreds of new books and magazines on Feng Shui. In our collective quest for health and happiness we are willing to consider pretty much anything – except attempting to understand our environment and to live in harmony with it. It is ironic that this unprecedented explosion of interest in Feng Shui has arisen after we have been living in a way that has broken all its rules.

KEEPING FIT

Exercise is an important part of health maintenance. The Far East is, of course, famous for the acrobatic feats of its martial artists. Less well known are what are called the 'internal' exercises, such as Tai Qi and Qi Gong. Their slow and gentle techniques belie their origins as true martial arts; generally, today it is only the meditation and health aspects that are taught. Both therapies are widely practised in China and it is common to see large numbers of people going through their daily routine in the open air each morning.

LEFT **Chinese acrobats, trained in martial arts, are renowned for their suppleness and strength.**

Tai Qi and Qi Gong

China's long history has been punctuated by war, invasion and occupation. At various times, occupying forces forbade the training of soldiers. However, clever generals worked round these rules to build an army by covert means. By slowing down the martial arts, they appeared to be harmless exercises. Soldiers could practise their fighting moves in secret. Weapons were also outlawed, so farm and agricultural tools were turned to militaristic uses. This can be seen today in many of the weapons used in martial arts, which have their origins in such devices as rice flails and scythes.

EXERCISES

The idea behind the internal exercises is that by strengthening the Qi of the body, illness can be avoided and body resistance strengthened. To learn Tai Qi or Qi Gong properly, you will need to find an experienced teacher. There are many different exercise routines and traditions within Tai Qi and Qi Gong, so teachers will vary significantly in their approach. All, however, will focus on helping you to control and strengthen your Qi. You can start by selecting the exercise that relates to your organ of weakness or Elemental type, and practise this daily.

ESSENTIALS
Tai Qi and Qi Gong are aimed at improving Qi management.

There are many traditional exercise routines, so classes can vary widely.

SPLEEN EXERCISE EARTH

1 Stand with your feet about shoulder-width apart, and knees slightly bent. Extend your arms in front of your stomach, palms facing downwards.

2 Inhale, moving your hands in a circle, ending above your head. Look upwards, and stretch. Keep your back straight.

3 With your knees slightly bent, exhale, and lower your arms to shoulder height. Return to the starting position. Perform the exercise ten times a day.

LUNG EXERCISE METAL

1 With your feet wide apart, extend your arms horizontally. Your palms should face down, with straight fingers.

2 Exhale, pulling your arms backwards and pushing out your chest. Inhale, returning your arms to the first position. Turn the palms upwards, curve the chest forwards, and rotate your arms clockwise. Repeat 20–30 times.

LIVER EXERCISE WOOD

1 This exercise also improves spinal mobility. Stand with your feet spread apart, and arms relaxed at your sides. Bend to the side and drop your arms down.

2 Start to draw a wide circle with your trunk and arms. Follow the circle round to the starting position. Keep your feet flat on the floor. Repeat the exercise ten times.

KIDNEY EXERCISE WATER

1 Stand with your hands on hips, feet about shoulder-width apart. Keep your legs as solid as possible, and bend from the waist.

2 Bend sideways, then forwards. This exercise represents the wind blowing through lotus leaves.

3 Finish by bending gently backwards. (Take great care if you have back problems.) Return to an upright position.

HEART EXERCISE FIRE

1 Stand with your feet slightly apart. Extend one arm in front of you, cupping the palm upwards. Raise the other arm, palm facing upwards, and stretch. Repeat with the opposite arms.

2 With palms facing the chest, lift your arms up with a strong movement, turning the palms to face upwards. Look to the sky, and hold the position. This exercise represents 'supporting the heavens'.

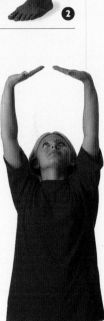

DIETARY MATTERS

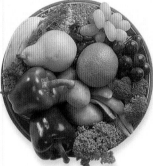

ABOVE **Vegetarianism is popular in the West, but virtually unknown in China.**

Chinese Medicine recommends a diet consisting mainly of fresh vegetables and grain (around 70 per cent), with small amounts of meat, fish, dairy products, nuts, seeds, fruits and pulses. Food traditions vary enormously across China, with hot spicy foods more popular in the colder provinces like Szechuan, while eggs and stirfries are associated with the hotter areas to the south.

Energy and flavour

The Chinese approach regards foods as containing either energy or flavour. Foods high in energy are light and revitalizing; bland grains and vegetables are examples. Flavour-rich foods are heavy and nourishing, and tend to be dense, wet, bloody or greasy. Examples of flavour-rich foods are animal products, rich grains, fruits and nuts.

We need both energy and flavour in our diet, but for good digestion we should eat more energy foods and fewer flavour foods. This is, of course, the opposite of what most of us prefer to do!

THE RAW AND THE COOKED

'Cooked food is not only tasty, but also greatly lessens the chance of catching disease, especially those of the digestive tract. Cooked food strengthens the body's resistance to disease, since the nutrients in the food are more readily digested and absorbed.' This quote comes from the writings of Zang Enquin, a master of Traditional Chinese Medicine.

LOOKING AFTER THE DIGESTION

The significance of raw and cooked food is vital in Chinese dietary theory. Raw food contains more nutrients than cooked food, as some nutrients are inevitably lost during cooking. However, Chinese Medicine believes that because cooked, warm food is so much more easily digested, there is an overall net gain in the nutrients the digestion can access. Therefore the amount of raw food eaten should be controlled, particularly in spring and summer, and consumed in relation to the current strength of the patient's digestion.

The process of digestion is like cooking a soup, which requires heat. Anything that is to be properly digested must be processed by the body at a temperature higher than normal body temperature. Therefore, it follows that well-chewed cooked food, rather than raw food, will require less energy from the body to digest. Chilling cooked food in the fridge, for reheating at a later point, can change its beneficial characteristics and warming abilities, so wherever possible eat freshly cooked meals.

Good habits

- Enjoy your food.
- Eat foods which are in season and grow locally.
- You should be relaxed and quiet while eating.
- Chew well.
- Eat until two-thirds full.
- Don't drink too much liquid while eating, especially cold drinks.
- Eat breakfast.
- Eat lunch.
- Don't eat late at night.
- Empty your bowels early in the morning.
- Eat according to your age, requirements, constitution and sex.

The digestive process

- Food is chopped up into small pieces by the teeth.
- In the Stomach, food is turned into a 'soup'.
- The soup is distilled into the Pure and the Impure.
- The Pure rises upwards to the Heart and Lungs.
- The Impure is excreted.
- The main food nutrients are turned into Blood and Qi.

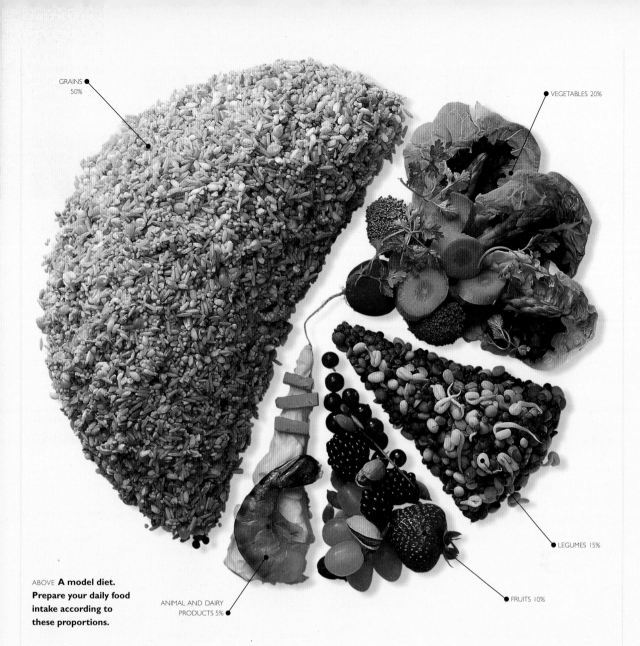

GRAINS
50%

VEGETABLES 20%

LEGUMES 15%

FRUITS 10%

ANIMAL AND DAIRY
PRODUCTS 5%

ABOVE **A model diet.
Prepare your daily food
intake according to
these proportions.**

Foods to avoid or
eat in limited amounts

- Milk
- Wheat
- Fried, barbecued
  or burnt food
- Foods fermented in
  vinegar or alcohol

- Coffee
- Sugar
- Polyunsaturated oils
- Animal fats
- Smoked or
  preserved meats

Good proportions

Your diet should be made up of different proportions of various
food groups. According to the principles of Chinese Medicine,
these are as follows:

GRAINS	50%
VEGETABLES	20%
LEGUMES (e.g. beans, peas, lentils, sprouted beans, soy products).	15%
FRUITS (including nuts and seeds).	15%
ANIMAL PRODUCTS (including dairy products).	5%

AVOIDING TOXINS

We live in an increasingly toxic world. It is probably now impossible to escape pollution, no matter where you live. The sources of toxic substances are so diverse that it can be hard to know how to start reducing your own exposure to them. There is undoubtedly a cumulative effect from toxins, so even though we cannot avoid them entirely, any reduction in exposure at home or work, and in the environment, is beneficial.

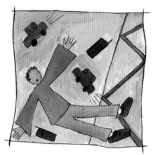

ABOVE **Toxins pervade everyday life: we are all affected by them.**

Toxin sources and how to avoid them

SOURCES IN THE HOME

GAS COOKERS
Harmful fumes are given off by the burning of domestic gas. These may be responsible for causing respiratory conditions.
✖ *Ventilate the kitchen well, or change your fuel source to electricity.*

PAINT FUMES
Paint gives off carcinogenic fumes for several days after application.
✖ *Ventilate the room thoroughly after you have painted it, and do not use it immediately. If the room is a bedroom, avoid sleeping in it for a few days.*

DIY SOLVENT PRODUCTS
Varnishes and glues give off harmful gases on application.
✖ *Wear a mask and gloves.*

MEDIUM DENSITY FIBREBOARD (MDF)
Formaldehyde is released by unsealed MDF for some time after manufacture. The fine dust created by sawing is a lung irritant.
✖ *Wear a mask when cutting MDF.*

CLEANING PRODUCTS
Dry-cleaning chemicals and products such as air-fresheners and bleach contain chemicals that may be carcinogenic.
✖ *Wear gloves and air clothes well.*

COSMETICS
The wood alcohol found in some cosmetics can damage cells.
✖ *Use as few cosmetics as possible, and buy from a natural products company.*

DENTAL AMALGAM FILLINGS
Mercury and other metals in fillings can leak into the body.
✖ *Consider having them replaced.*

CENTRAL HEATING
Dry air damages the lungs.
✖ *Use humidifiers, or other heat sources.*

DOUBLE GLAZING
A contained atmosphere traps pathogens in the house.
✖ *Open the windows.*

FITTED CARPETS
Provide a home for dust-mites.
✖ *Change to wood floors and rugs.*

FOOD SOURCES

PESTICIDE RESIDUES
Most crops are grown with pesticides which affect the immune system, and which are not removed by water alone.
✖ *Wash fruit and vegetables well in soapy water. Alternatively, choose organically grown produce.*

PRESERVATIVES, COLOURINGS AND E NUMBERS
Implicated in a wide range of illnesses, including hyperactivity.
✖ *Avoid.*

STIMULANTS
Alcohol, coffee, tobacco and recreational drugs deplete the immune system, causing illness.
✖ *Minimize your intake, or cut them out of your life completely.*

HIDDEN SUGARS
High in calories and bad for teeth.
✖ *Read the labels on foods, looking for things such as fructose and glucose, and avoid these products.*

TRANS FATTY ACIDS (TFAS)

Highly saturated fats found in margarines or convenience foods.
✖ *Avoid.*

ANTIBIOTICS IN MEAT

Adds to the overuse of antibiotics, depleting the immune system.
✖ *Eat organic meat.*

BURNT, RANCID, OLD, PRESERVED OR LEFTOVER FOOD

Devoid of nutrition and may be carcinogenic or toxic.
✖ *Avoid.*

GENETICALLY ENGINEERED FOOD

This is a recent innovation which has not been thoroughly tested.
✖ *Eat organic food.*

AT WORK

PHOTOCOPIERS/FAXES/MOBILE PHONES/COMPUTERS

Electronic radiation is implicated as a cause of cancer.
✖ *Place plants on or next to your desk.*

AIR-CONDITIONING

Transmits viruses and bacteria.
✖ *Don't sit underneath the vents.*

DRINKS VENDING MACHINES

The drinks contain unknown ingredients.
✖ *Make your own drinks.*

STRESS

Attacks the immune system.
✖ *Practise relaxation techniques.*

SYNTHETIC OFFICE FURNISHINGS

Emit poisonous gases.
✖ *Move to an eco-friendly employer.*

VDU RADIATION EMISSIONS

There is no safe level of exposure to radiation.
✖ *Use a radiation screen.*

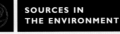

SOURCES IN THE ENVIRONMENT

POLLUTION FROM TRANSPORT

Carbon monoxide, toxic airborne particles and volatile organic compounds (VOCs) are pumped out by petrol-powered vehicles. Children are particularly susceptible to them.
✖ *Don't add to environmental pollution. Use a car only when really necessary. Walk, take public transport, or cycle – make sure you wear a mask.*

PETROL/DIESEL GASES

A strong, direct pollution source.
✖ *Avoid breathing in vapour while filling your tank.*

CONTAMINATED WATER

Tap water may contain toxins; plastic bottles may contain the residues of solvents.
✖ *Drink filtered or bottled water (preferably from glass bottles).*

PHARMACEUTICALS

The unnecessary use of medical drugs, particularly antibiotics, weakens the body's response to outside attack.
✖ *Only use antibiotics when essential; practise preventative medicine.*

POWER CABLES/POWER STATIONS

Strong radiation, which may cause illness, is present at these sites.
✖ *Move house.*

NATURAL UNDERGROUND GASES SUCH AS RADON

Radon is known to cause cancer.
✖ *Move house.*

OZONE

Holes in the ozone layer cause more skin cancers to develop.
✖ *Wear sunblock and a hat.*

CHLOROFLUOROCARBONS (CFCS)

Deplete the ozone layer; are involved in complex chemical reactions that are harmful.
✖ *Ensure that your fridge, and any household aerosols you use, are CFC-free.*

PETS

Animals play host to a range of pests and pathogens.
✖ *Avoid animals if you are sensitive to them. Protect pets against parasites.*

PARASITES, MICRO-ORGANISMS AND VIRUSES

Responsible for allergies, auto-immune and digestive disorders.
✖ *Strengthen your immune system. Take care when travelling abroad.*

Supplementation

Certain foods, vitamins and minerals contain natural antioxidants that protect the body against cancer.

Regular, long-term consumption of these nutrients can reduce your chances of developing cancer.

GREEN TEA

SELENIUM. FOUND IN BRAZIL NUTS

VITAMINS A, C, E; CO-ENZYME Q10

BARLEY (DO NOT USE IF PREGNANT) AND WHEAT GRASS

OMEGA-3 AND OMEGA-6 FATTY ACIDS (FOUND IN FISH OILS, OLIVE, SESAME, WALNUT, FLAX AND HEMP OILS)

FRESH SPROUTED PLANTS SUCH AS BEAN AND SEED SPROUTS

HOW A CHINESE PHYSICIAN WORKS

Going to see a traditional Chinese physician is usually a very different experience from consulting an orthodox doctor, both in terms of what the consultation involves and the basis of the approach. A whole-body medical system works on two levels: the physician is dealing with the problem the patient is presenting, while at the same time looking for potential problems that might occur in the future.

ABOVE **Chinese physicians look at multiple aspects of your health to head off future problems.**

The physician

BELOW **The information you volunteer, and the way that you present it, gives the physician a good insight into your condition before the physical examination takes place.**

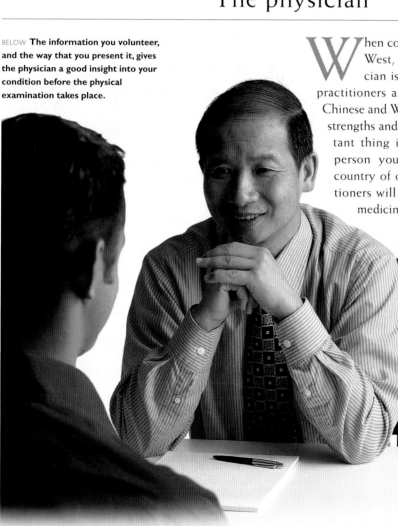

When consulting a Chinese physician in the West, you may well find that the physician is not from China. The majority of practitioners are Europeans or Americans. Both Chinese and Western practitioners have their own strengths and weaknesses. Essentially, the important thing is that you get on well with the person you are consulting, irrespective of country of origin. All properly trained practitioners will have learnt enough conventional medicine to understand your problem from the perspective of an orthodox doctor. Their therapeutic approaches will also vary – some may use only herbs, others will add acupuncture, cupping, massage or Qi Gong.

Treating a disease once symptoms have occurred is like digging a well when thirsty.

TRADITIONAL
CHINESE SAYING

BELOW **Your physician will be able to collect a lot of information from your pulse alone.**

FEELING THE QUALITY OF THE QI

MERIDIAN

The number of times you will need to see the physician will vary depending on the severity of the condition, the length of time you have had it, and your general health and constitution. It is impossible to generalize, but it's likely that a problem with very extreme symptoms, which you have had for most of your life, will take a considerable time to respond fully.

NATURAL MEDICINES

Remember that natural medicines work in a very different fashion to orthodox Western drugs and treatment. Herbs, acupuncture and dietary therapy stimulate your body's own mechanisms, bringing about a state of balance by creating internal harmony. Drugs and surgical methods inhibit or suppress a particular symptom or reaction in the body, thus stopping the symptoms from being apparent. There is no doubt that modern medicine works faster and often more powerfully than traditional medicine, but you must weigh up the long-term effects of such treatments.

WHAT HAPPENS DURING A CONSULTATION?

The procedure that you will encounter at a first appointment will follow a broadly similar pattern, although there can be variations.

First, information is gathered by asking questions. This is to get the details of the background to the problem, but also gives the physician the opportunity to see how you present yourself, hear your tone of voice, and gauge your mental state.

At some point your tongue will be examined and your pulse checked. The physician may also palpate the abdomen, or check a relevant part of the body. Although tests such as measuring blood-pressure are not part of a traditional diagnosis, you may find that these are carried out if they are thought to be necessary.

TREATMENT

By putting all this information together, a unique picture of your health is produced, where any disease is revealed as a pattern of disharmony. This diagnosis points to the type of treatment required to address the problem and set you on the path to recovery.

BELOW **Analysing the appearance of your tongue gives as much information as a body scan.**

ESSENTIALS
Find a physician who you like and trust, regardless of their nationality.

Sometimes herbs work quickly and dramatically, but more often treatment is lengthy.

BELOW **You may be prescribed a decoction, tincture, pills or another herbal remedy.**

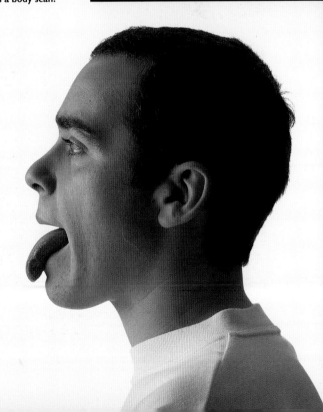

WHEN TO CONSULT A PHYSICIAN

Health maintenance is a daily activity which includes proper diet, regular exercise and stress management. It can also include the diagnosing and treatment of problems, and this is the aim of this book. However, it is vital that we should know when to consult an expert. There will be times in all our lives when it is critical to seek the guidance of an experienced physician in order to return us to a state of good health.

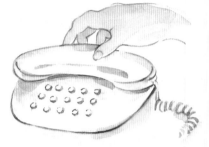

ABOVE **Get professional help if you are not making any headway with your health problem.**

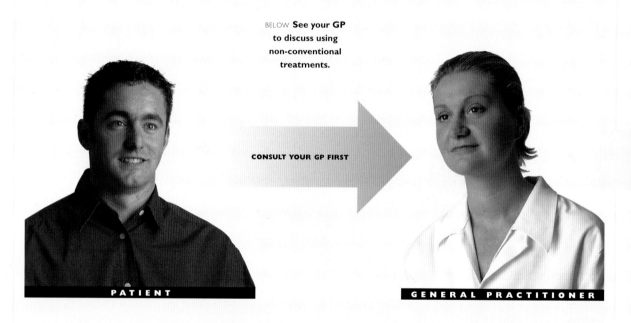

BELOW **See your GP to discuss using non-conventional treatments.**

CONSULT YOUR GP FIRST

PATIENT

GENERAL PRACTITIONER

Professional help

The most obvious examples of times when it is necessary to consult a professional are cases of life-threatening or serious illness, or when pregnant. However, even general chronic complaints may require additional assistance if your own efforts at self-medication are not producing results.

Consulting an orthodox doctor does not necessarily rule out non-conventional treatments, as many doctors will recommend non-conventional treatments in addition to conventional drugs. If you intend to see several specialists, it is important for a single professional, perhaps your GP, to co-ordinate the recommendations and treatments from the other practitioners. For you to derive the maximum benefit, the treatments must work in harmony. In rare cases herbal remedies can interfere with orthodox drugs, so ensure that your herbalist and GP are aware of all the remedies or drugs you are taking.

FINDING A CHINESE HERBALIST

The availability of properly trained physicians in your area will vary enormously depending on where you live. Most countries now have a professional association for Chinese herbalists. These organizations will have a set of criteria that members must meet, and will usually require professional insurance and adherence to a code of ethics. There will be a complaints procedure to use if you are unhappy about the treatment you have received from one of their members.

I strongly recommend that you only consult a physician who is a member of the professional body in your country, or it will be impossible to gauge the authenticity of their qualifications.

ACUPUNCTURIST

ABOVE **Acupuncture offers an alternative for certain problems.**

QUESTIONS TO ASK

When you have selected a physician, contact him or her before making an initial appointment. Ask whether the physician has had any experience of your particular problem, and how it might be treated.

There is little point in asking how much treatment will be required, as it will be almost impossible to gauge this until a full case history has been taken. You should also ask about fees.

HOW FAR DO I TRAVEL?

Try and see someone who is reasonably near you, if at all possible. It is not uncommon for people to travel halfway across a country, even to a different country, to see a famous physician that they have heard of. This is often counterproductive. The additional stress and expense of travelling, and the long periods between appointments, will usually outweigh the confidence that you have placed in the physician. This course of action is probably only worthwhile if your condition is rare and especially difficult to treat.

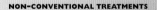

NON-CONVENTIONAL TREATMENTS

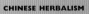

CHINESE HERBALISM

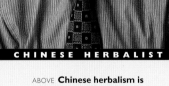

CHINESE HERBALIST

ABOVE **Chinese herbalism is suitable for everybody, from the young to the old.**

You may prefer to go and see someone who has been recommended by a friend or relative, which is a good way of finding a practitioner. However, you should still establish that this person is a registered practitioner. Be wary of people who say that they do not need to be a member of any professional organization.

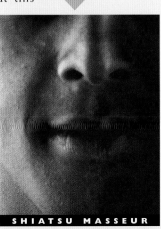

RIGHT **Shiatsu restores the flow of Qi within the body by massage.**

SHIATSU MASSEUR

ESSENTIALS

Keep your GP or other key practitioner fully aware of all treatments and medication that you are trying.

Choose a practitioner who has some experience of your problem. Ask plenty of questions about what will be involved.

GLOSSARY

Allopathy: the treatment of disease by conventional means, common in the West, using drugs which have opposite effects to the disease symptoms.

Blood: a concept embracing all the moistening, nourishing and cooling processes in the body. Particularly important to women's health.

Cold: a Yin influence causing understimulation.

Confucius (551–479 BC): ancient Chinese scholar famous for his *Analects*, the posthumously-published collection of his sayings and teachings, and for codifying the *I Ching*.

Congee: traditional Chinese rice porridge.

Damp, Dampness: abnormal body fluids which become thick and cause disharmony and disease.

Damp-Cold: combined Cold and Dampness with the characteristics of both.

Damp-Heat: combined Heat and Dampness with the characteristics of both.

Decoction: a method for preparing herbs, involving simmering them in boiling water for an hour or more.

Deficiency: a weakness – in an organ, of the Blood or of the Qi – which results in disharmony.

Detoxification: the process of clearing toxins from the body by careful dieting and intake of fluids.

Dryness: a lack of Yin leading to an absence, or lack of, fluid.

Eight Principles (or Eight Conditions): four pairs of opposites – Yin-Yang, Full-Empty, Interior-Exterior and Heat-Cold – which are used to describe medical conditions.

Empty, Emptiness (Xu): the lack of a particular substance in the body, leading to a disharmony.

Empty-Cold: Cold due to a lack of Yang.

Empty-Heat: Heat due to a lack of Yin.

Exterior: an imbalance arising from an external cause.

Feng Shui (*feng* meaning wind, *shui* meaning water): the practice of siting buildings and objects with regard to the influences of natural surroundings.

Fire: an extreme form of Heat. Also one of the Five Elements, symbolizing joy, fulfillment and happiness.

Five Elements: a way of categorizing natural energies, and of describing forces within the body. The Five Elements are Earth, Metal, Wood, Water and Fire.

Five Flavours: the tastes (sweet, sour, bitter, salty and pungent) associated with the Five Elements.

Five Seasons: winter, summer, spring, autumn and the transitional season which occurs between each. Each season is related to an element.

Full, Fullness (Shi): an excess of a particular substance in the body, leading to a disharmony.

Full-Cold: Cold due to too much Yin.

Full-Heat: Heat due to too much Yang.

Heat: a Yang influence causing over-stimulation.

Holism: a branch of medicine which treats the whole person, taking mental and social factors into account, rather than just the disease.

Huang Di (the Yellow Emperor, 259–210 BC): founder of the Qin dynasty. Author of the *Nei Jing Su Wen*, the *Classic of Internal Medicine*, along with his physician Qi Bo.

I Ching (or *Yi Jing – Book of Changes*): a divination text, one of the fundamental texts of Chinese philosophy.

Infusion: a method of taking herbs, involving pouring boiling water directly onto dried herbs and straining the mixture almost immediately.

Interior: an imbalance arising from an internal cause.

Jin Ye: body fluids, including Blood and Phlegm.

Jing, or Inherited Qi: the Qi we are born with, and which determines our basic constitution.

Li Shi Zhen: Chinese physician responsible for the ancient text *Classic of the Pulse*.

Mao Tse Dong (1893–1976): Chinese leader (1935–1976) and first Chairman of the People's Republic. Famous for his political philosophy as set out in the *Little Red Book*. During his Cultural Revolution, much traditional knowledge of Chinese Medicine was lost.

Meridians: the pathways in the human body through which Qi flows; used in acupuncture.

Palpation: the practice of using the fingers and hand to touch a part of the body in order to discover any disharmonies which may be affecting it.

Patent remedies: herbal medicines ready-prepared and sold over the counter by herbalists.

Phlegm: mucus which has become pathological through the action of Stagnant Damp, or from the action of Heat and Cold on normal mucus.

Qi: the life force – natural energy present in all living things. Qi which is blocked or stagnant may cause pain or disease.

Qi Gong: a gentle martial art, composed of breathing, meditation and movement, aimed at directing the Qi.

San Jiao: Triple Heater, one of the Twelve Organs.

Shen: the mind or spirit. Said to reside in the Heart.

Shen Nong (the Divine Farmer): mythical figure believed to have taught mankind how to grow food and herbs, and credited with introducing the art of herbalism to the Chinese.

Shi: see Full.

Shiatsu: a vigorous form of massage designed to stimulate the Qi.

Six Evils: external causes of illness. The Six Evils are: Wind, Cold, Fire, Summer Heat, Dryness and Damp.

Stagnation: a condition arising from a blockage of the Qi. Most commonly seen in Food Stagnation, wherein overeating or a bad diet will result in digestive disorders; or in Qi Stagnation, which is believed to give rise to pain.

Tai Qi: a gentle martial art.

Taoism: Chinese philosophy advocating humility and religious piety.

Tincture: a method of preparing herbs, involving soaking them in alcohol.

Twelve Organs/Twelve Officials: the term for the anatomical organs which Chinese Medicine considers to be the most important – the Heart, Spleen, Liver, Lungs, Kidneys, Large Intestine, Small Intestine, Triple Heater, Bladder, Gall Bladder, Pericardium and Stomach – and their associated functions and responsibilities.

Wind: a concept embracing movement, and also the idea of disease carried through the air. Is generally thought to be a malign influence, and is one of the External Evils. It may be retained in the body and cause allergies or disharmonies.

Xin Bao: Pericardium, one of the Twelve Organs.

Xu: see Empty.

Yin-Yang: the idea that everything is based on pairs of opposing forces, and that healthy living depends on keeping the opposing forces well-balanced. Yin (dark, cool, calm, downwards, passivity, moisture) and Yang (light, warm, active, upwards, dryness) are relative terms; everything contains aspects of both Yin and Yang.

Zangfu system: ten of the Twelve Organs – excluding the Triple Heater and the Pericardium – each of which are either Yin or Yang, and have an affinity to one of the Five Elements.

SUPPLIERS

There are a number of different ways in which you can get the herbs you may need for self-treatment.

FROM A HERBAL PHYSICIAN

As I discuss on *pages 178–181*, I strongly recommend that you find a registered herbalist with whom you can build a relationship; this is the best way of ensuring your long-term health and welfare. Your physician will be able to prescribe the herbs you need and advise on your self-treatment. As a registered practitioner, they will have access to good quality, authentic herbs. Only ever consult a physician who is registered with the professional body for your country. For the UK and Ireland, these are:

THE REGISTER OF CHINESE HERBAL MEDICINE

PO Box 400, Wembley

Middlesex, HA9 9NZ

Tel: 0171 224 0803

www.rchm.co.uk

THE NATIONAL INSTITUTE OF MEDICAL HERBALISTS

56 Longbrook Street

Exeter, Devon, EX4 6AH

Tel: 01392 426022

When requesting information from these organizations, it is always a good idea to include a large stamped, self-addressed envelope and a donation of around £2–£3.

FROM A HEALTH SHOP

There are a variety of shops offering health foods and herbal products. Small, specialized stores will often have a more personalized service and the person behind the counter will usually be knowledgeable about their products. Health shops are a good source of simple, single-herb products, especially those containing Western herbs. Most often, the herbs will come packaged as tinctures or pills. Make sure that you seek advice before purchasing products containing a combination of herbs or vitamins.

FROM A CHEMIST

Most chemists and pharmacies now stock a range of herbal and natural products. However, staff are not usually specifically trained in this area and are unlikely to be able to offer you much advice.

FROM THE INTERNET

I would strongly advise against purchasing herbal products through the internet, as it is impossible to obtain assurances about the quality of the herbs, and the accountability or authenticity of the supplier.

FROM CHINESE SUPERMARKETS

Most Chinese supermarkets will stock a few bags of dried herbs and some popular pill formulas; they also often stock soup mixes of dried herbs which are added to food as a tonic. However, the quality of the herbs is variable, and they are often rather expensive. Prepared remedies will often combine Western allopathic drugs with herbs, which is illegal in this country.

FROM A CHINESE PHARMACY

There has been an explosion of Chinese herb shops in the West over the last few years, and most large towns will now have one. However, be aware that it is impossible for the lay person to distinguish a properly-trained Chinese Medicine practitioner from an amateur; an array of certificates on the wall is not a guarantee of authenticity. The only way to be sure that you are consulting a proper physician is to contact the professional body in your country (see above).

THROUGH NETWORK MARKETING

There are an increasing number of companies selling herbal products through network marketing (a term for pyramid selling), particularly in the USA. The products themselves are usually of a good quality, but they are almost always strongly-branded pre-packaged combinations which make it hard for you to tailor your medicine to suit your own pattern.

FURTHER READING

If you would like to learn about Chinese Medicine in more detail, here are some suggestions for books which would help to develop your knowledge.

THE WEB THAT HAS NO WEAVER
Ted Kaptchuck
Congdon and Weed, 1983

THE CHINESE WAY TO HEALTH:
A SELF-HELP GUIDE TO TRADITIONAL CHINESE MEDICINE
Dr Stephen Gascoigne
Charles E Tuttle Co, 1983

HEALING WITH WHOLE FOODS:
ORIENTAL TRADITIONS AND MODERN NUTRITION
Paul Pitchford
Atlantic Books, 1996

THE TAO OF HEALTHY EATING:
DIETARY WISDOM ACCORDING TO TRADITIONAL CHINESE MEDICINE
Bob Flaws
Blue Poppy Press, 1998

A HISTORY OF CHINESE MEDICINE
Dominique Hoizey and Marie-Joseph Hoizey, translated by Paul Bailey.
This title is now out of print, but copies should be available in larger libraries.

UNDERSTANDING THE I CHING:
THE WILHELM LECTURES ON THE BOOK OF CHANGES (MYTHOS)
Hellmut Willhelm and Richard Willhelm, translated by CF Baynes
Princeton University Press, 1995
There are literally hundreds of versions of the *I Ching* available in English (not to mention those available in Chinese!); this is the one I would most recommend.

THE NEW HOLISTIC HERBAL
David Hoffman
Element Books, 1991

BETWEEN HEAVEN AND EARTH:
A GUIDE TO CHINESE MEDICINE
Harriet Benfield and Efrem Korngold
Ballantine Books, 1992

INDEX

HERB INDEX

ACKNOWLEDGEMENTS

The publishers would like to thank the following for the use of pictures:

The Hutchison Library: p 42 (l) (John Wright), p 172 (tl) (Melanie Friend)
The Image Bank, London: p 14 (tl), p50
Rex Features, London: p 84 (r)
The Stock Market Photo Agency: p 14 (tr), p 26 (bl), p 29 (b), p 44 (b), p 45 (t), p 48, p 49, p 74 (tl), p 81,
p 82 (r), p 86 (t), p 93, p 114 (l), p 142 (l), p 169 (bl), p 170 (tl)
The Science Photo Library: p 16 (tl), p 64 (bl), p 144 (tl)
Wellcome Institute Library: p 52 (t), p 162 (tl)

The publishers would like to thank the following for help with photography:

Helen Furbear
Mayway (UK) Company Ltd
Western Herbs